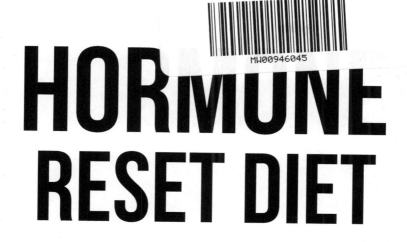

HORMONE RESET DIET

*Balance Hormones, Recharge Health and
Lose Weight Effortlessly!*

HORMONE RESET DIET RECIPES INCLUDED!

VALERIE CHILDS

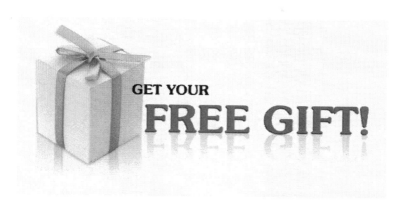

WAIT! – DO YOU LIKE FREE BOOKS?

My **FREE Gift** to You!! As a way to say **Thank You** for downloading my book, I'd like to offer you more **FREE BOOKS!** Each time we release a NEW book, we offer it first to a small number of people as a test - drive. Because of your commitment here in downloading my book, I'd love for you to be a part of this group. You can join easily here → http://smoothieslimdown.com/

Table of Contents

Introduction

H ey there! Thank you for picking up this book!

You and I, as well as the dozens of other women who also made the conscious decision to take action against their weight gain through this book, have something in common – you've experienced how difficult it is to lose weight after several *(and I do mean several)* diet and exercise attempts.

Weight loss has probably been the oldest struggle in the book for the majority of the female population. Book after book has been released, claiming to be the true cure for fat and obesity, but only a few really deliver what they promised. Is it because the book programs weren't effective? Is it because the dieting and exercising programs found in these books weren't done properly? Or is it because numerous authors have overlooked one, single factor that may have appeared trivial but, in truth, has been the culprit for women's mood swings, changing bodily functions, abnormal eating habits and slowed metabolism?

Personally, I'm betting my money on the last question and you should too. Hormones have never really been the core topic for a weight loss book because, even though, medically, they have been known to affect weight under certain circumstances, they weren't viewed as a major player, unlike eating right *(dieting)* and training your body *(exercising)*.

This is exactly what we're going to explore in this book! Hormones may not have been key topics in several weight loss books but, now, we're going to get to the bottom of how you can beat flab by resetting your hormones. We're also going to learn more about the different processes and recipes involved in Hormone Reset and it doesn't stop there.

Get excited because this book might just be the very thing you've been waiting for!

Chapter 1

YOU AND YOUR HORMONES

Before we go to the good stuff, let's first understand the facts. When a woman's hormones are out of sync, it can lead to several effects on our body, which includes the build-up of fat. If you have extra handles on you, chances are, you have one or two of the following hormonal imbalances:

➤ High Estrogen

➤ Low Testosterone

➤ High Insulin

➤ High Cortisol

➤ High Leptin

➤ Deficient Growth Hormone

➤ Deficient Thyroid Hormone

Estrogen

Estrogen and fat have a very complicated relationship. Fat isn't just a big blob of lard sitting on your hips. It's a vital part of your hormone system since one of its major jobs is to produce estrogen. An enzyme called aromatase contained in fat tissues converts testosterone to estrogen. There are loads more where estrogen came from. This is just one source of it that's important to know in weight loss/weight gain situations.

It can also work the other way around. Estrogen overload can exaggerate hypothyroid issues, slowing down your metabolism and causing you to gain weight. Another possibility is that high levels of estrogen promote fat gain through the prevention of using these fats as energy.

Like what I said, it's a complicated relationship but more certain than not, estrogen is a key hormone to weight gain or weight loss.

(source: Paleoleap)

Testosterone

Testosterone is a hormone found in both men and women. It's the hormone responsible for increased muscle mass, bone density and metabolism. A low level of testosterone can lead to an increased risk for depression, low sex drive, obesity and osteoporosis.

(source: LiveStrong)

Insulin

Here's how the normal process goes: after we eat our bodies release insulin which tells our muscles, livers and fat cells to take up the sugar and fat and remove it from our bloodstream since it could be toxic for the body. However, the liver and muscle cells have a limited capacity to store glucose (*or sugar*) hence they shut their "doors" when excessive carbs are consumed on a daily basis even with the pancreas releasing enough amounts of insulin. Having nowhere else to go, the sugar in our blood gets sent to fat cells. The result? I think you know...

With the "doors" shut, the pancreas will release more insulin to normalize blood sugar levels. With more insulin released, glucose levels can be brought down to a safe level again...at least for a while. Over time, fasting blood sugar levels start to creep up and the entire process will result to insulin resistance.

(source: LifeTime-WeightLoss)

Cortisol

When we're stressed, several hormones are released. This includes adrenalin, which gives us instant energy, corticotrophin releasing hormone or CRH and cortisol. Adrenalin and CRH, at high levels, cause a decrease in appetite. This effect, however, doesn't usually last very long. Cortisol, on the other hand, works in a very different way. Its main function is to help our body replenish after the stress has gone. It "hangs around" a bit longer and elevated levels of this cause an increase in our appetite, driving us to eat more.

(source: WebMD)

Leptin

Leptin is another hormone secreted by fat cells. Its main role is to send signals to the brain, telling it that our bodies have enough energy stored up and that we don't need to eat. If you have increased amounts of this, your brain should be telling your body that it's had enough, right? Yes, that is what's supposed to happen. In the case of obesity, an increased leptin has been found in the bloodstream but the problem is the brain doesn't recognize it. This state is called leptin resistance.

But, why in the world is our brain blinded when insane amounts of leptin are already in our body? It's because of another hormone called insulin. It could be one of the reasons why our brain is not picking up on the signal leptin is giving off. Darn you insulin!

FUN FACT: No matter how strong your will power is, it will not work if you have leptin resistance. This just goes to show that you cannot go against nature *(or against the reactions of your body)*.

(source: AuthorityNutrition)

Growth Hormone

Isn't growth hormone supposed to make you grow? So, low levels of it will make you small?

Yes, generally, that's the idea. Children with a growth hormone deficiency are, generally, smaller than their peers but it isn't only the growth that it's responsible for. One of its functions is to regulate our bodies' metabolism. Adults with a deficiency have been found to have high levels of fat as well as cholesterol in their bodies. Many would link this to unhealthy eating but even if an adult eat well but has ADGH *(Adult Growth Hormone Deficiency)*, similar findings will be observed.

(source: HealthLine)

Thyroid Hormone

Thyroid hormones also play a major role in our body in connection with weight loss or weight gain. One of its functions is to, basically, regulate our calorie intake. A deficiency in this hormone results in a low basal metabolic rate and a difficulty to lose extra weight. Sounds familiar to you?

(source: Women to Women)

There are more…

It doesn't stop there too. This is just an overview of the many hormones involved in the process of weight gain. Am I saying that there are more hormones and not just the seven already mentioned? YES.

The whole thing sounds so alarming, doesn't it? "What other hormones are out of whack in my body?" you might be asking but don't go running to your doctor to get some tests done just yet.

Hormonal imbalances, though very scientific sounding, are not medical issues but, more often, they are a nutritional issue.

It is true and it is surprising. The very thing that you're snacking on right now may be causing your body, as well as your hormones, to go crazy on food. So, put the snack down slowly and let's continue.

I'm saying this not because I want to scare you to do a Hormone Reset *(well, maybe I am just a little)* but I'm saying this so your eyes can be opened to the facts. It isn't only diet and exercises that will help us lose a couple of pounds. They're good on their own but the idea that I want to leave you is this:

A more effective approach to weight loss is by controlling or managing the very things that affect the inside of our body – these are hormones.

Chapter 2

WHAT IS HORMONE RESET?

Did I tickle your interest yet? If you've gone this far, maybe I have and that's a good thing. Now that we know the facts *(the ugly truth so to speak)*, let's take a look at what hormone reset is.

So we already talked about "going against nature" with will power, diets and exercises, right? Though these may be effective, we still go through a lot just to maintain whatever we have going on.

For example, let's say you were on a diet. One night, you craved something sugary or something salty. You resist the urge *(though very difficult for you)*. Your stomach, however, has other plans and it's not letting you forget about your craving. Eventually, a couple of nights with this episode, you're bound to give in. That's why a lot of people have cheat days! You probably have one yourself or maybe everyday is a cheat day.

Sooner or later, nature will win because that's just how our body works – or doesn't work, in this case because of our broken metabolism caused by hormonal imbalances.

Hormone Reset is aimed at correcting this. It is a form of a diet and you would need to exercise your will power during the first few tries but, eventually, you'll ease in to it and you'll get the hang of it because you're managing what goes on inside your body rather than controlling outside factors.

Chapter 3

WHY SHOULD YOU AND I RESET OUR HORMONES?

OK so you're probably skeptical and you're asking me this question. You're asking me for reasons why you, or anyone else for that matter, need to reset their hormones.

Fair enough and I have just the answers for your question:

1. You (and many others like you) need a change.

If you're tired of doing diet after diet, and exercise after exercise without getting the results you're expecting, then what have you got to lose? You need a change and this could be it.

2. Your body needs it.

I can't stress this enough. The main reason why many diets and exercises fail is because they've neglected one big factor and that's hormones. Learning how to control your hormones will give you a new perspective on how your body works. And, knowing how your body works will give you fresher ideas on how you can keep it healthy.

3. You'll feel loads better about yourself.

I know that exercise also promises the same thing with the release of endorphins (*the happy hormone*) but that's just one. Imagine how fabulous you're going to feel if you've reset all the six hormones we're focusing on.

4. You'll lose weight (almost effortlessly).

This is our main goal, right? Aside from being healthy and being educated on how your body works, you'll also lose weight, which is what we're all trying to do!

Because you are targeting what's happening on the inside of your body, you're not going against any natural reaction with will power. All you really need is to cook the suggested recipes and eat!

Chapter 4

GETTING READY FOR HORMONE RESET DIET

Now to the meat of this book! Enough about all these talks of facts and fundamentals; let's, now, talk about how we can prep ourselves for Hormone Reset.

The Way it Works

You will be doing resets 3 days at a time. There are 7 hormones to focus on and you will be resetting one after another for 3 days, which is the minimum amount of time needed to reset a metabolic hormone. You'll start by eliminating meat, then sugar, fruit, caffeine, moving on to grain, dairy and then, last but not least, toxins.

Base Measurements

To start, you're going to have to have metrics to measure against so you'll know if you've, indeed, improved or not *(it's highly likely that you will, though)*. These metrics would include:

- Body mass index

- Basal metabolic rate

- Sleep

- Blood pressure

- Blood sugar

- Body fat

- Body measurements *(like your waist, arms, legs, etc)*

Acquiring these measurements is simple. You can ask your family doctor to help you out, you can do it yourself *(for some like blood pressure and body measurements)* and, lastly, you can make use of online resources, which can help you measure your Basal metabolic rate and body mass index.

When you're done, the next step is to plan your meals and do a bit of grocery shopping.

What to Do Exactly

Since you know that you're eliminating certain foods in your diet 3 days at a time, all you need to do is keep in mind what needs to be eliminated.

For example, 1st 3 days = no red meat.

1. The day before you start, choose the meals that appeal to you the most on the recipes section under "No to Red Meat". Once you've chosen, shop for 3 days worth of ingredients.

2. When day 1 comes, prepare your breakfast, lunch and dinner respectively and maybe you can throw in a bit of snacks in between.

3. Go through your meals for the entire 3 days and then move on the next which reset, which is no sugar.

Go through the process until you've completely reset all 7 metabolic hormones.

Tips to Remember

✓ If you're a busy person, and I'm sure you are, make sure to do advanced preparations for your meals. Marinate what needs to be marinated, chop what needs to be chopped and so on. This way, when time comes to actually cook your meals, all you have to do is to assemble the ingredients and cook them together.

✓ As mentioned earlier, you'll be exercising a certain amount of will power in the beginning so make sure that you do. Because we are eliminating certain foods in your diet, your body may experience cravings. Don't worry because it gets easier. Trust me!

✓ Don't be scared to customize. You already have the basic idea: 1st 3 days = no red meat; 2nd 3 days = no fruit and so on. Don't be afraid to add in personal recipes in your breakfast, lunch or dinner. The recipes found in this book merely serve as a guide. The more you put your personal touch on this program, the more chances you have of really claiming success.

✓ Keep a record handy. In the midst of your busy day, you might forget that you're on a no fruit diet. To remind you, keep a note on your phone or set your phone to alarm every eating time. You can also have a journal to inspire you more on your journey.

Chapter 5

HORMONE RESET RECIPES

"No to Red Meat" Recipes

B y eliminating red meat and alcohol in our diet, we're resetting the hormone estrogen.

The Really Good Veggie Meatloaf

INGREDIENTS	NUTRITION FACTS (Per Serving)	
2 cups water	✓ Calories	264
1 teaspoon salt	✓ Calories from Fat 92	35%
1 cup lentils	✓ Total Fat 10.2g	15%
1 small onion, diced	✓ Saturated Fat 5.2g	26%
1 cup quick-cooking oats	✓ Cholesterol 69.1mg	23%
3⁄4 cup grated cheddar cheese	✓ Sodium 810.4mg	33%
or 3⁄4 cup Swiss cheese, cheese	✓ Total Carbohydrate 29g	9%
or 3⁄4 cup Monterey jack cheese	✓ Dietary Fiber 7g	27%
or 3⁄4 cup American cheese	✓ Sugars 3.6g	14%
1 egg, beaten	✓ Protein 14.8g	29%
4 1⁄2 ounces spaghetti sauce or		
4 1⁄2 ounces tomato sauce		
1 teaspoon garlic powder		
1 teaspoon dried basil		
1 tablespoon dried parsley		
1⁄2 teaspoon seasoning salt		
1⁄4 teaspoon black pepper		
6 SERVINGS		
TOTAL TIME 85MINS		

Instructions:

1. Add salt to water and boil in a saucepan.

2. Add lentils and simmer covered 25-30 minutes, until lentils are soft and most of water is evaporated.

3. Remove from fire.

4. Drain and partially mash lentils.

5. Scrape into mixing bowl and allow to cool slightly.

6. Stir in onion, oats and cheese until mixed.

7. Add egg, tomato sauce, garlic, basil, parsley, seasoning salt and pepper.

8. Mix well.

9. Spoon into loaf pan that has been generously sprayed with Pam (non-stick cooking spray) or well greased.

10. Smooth top with back of spoon.

11. Bake at 350 degrees for 30- 45 minutes until top of loaf is dry, firm and golden brown.

12. Cool in pan on rack for about 10 minutes.

13. Run a sharp knife around edges of pan then turn out loaf onto serving platter.

Lime Spiced Grilled Chicken

INGREDIENTS	NUTRITION FACTS (Per Serving)	
6 boneless skinless chicken breast halves	✓ Calories 50	
2 cloves garlic (minced)	✓ Calories from Fat 40	
2 tbsps extra-virgin olive oil		
2 tbsps lime juice (freshly squeezed)	**% Daily Value ***	
2 tsps onion powder	✓ Total Fat 4.5g	7%
2 tsps lime zest (freshly grated)	✓ Saturated Fat 0.5g	3%
1 tsp oregano (chopped)	✓ Trans Fat	
1 tsp red pepper flakes	✓ Cholesterol	0%
kosher salt	✓ Sodium 135mg	6%
freshly ground pepper	✓ Potassium 50mg	1%
	✓ Total Carbohydrate 3g	1%
6 SERVINGS	✓ Dietary Fiber	
TOTAL TIME 45MINS	less than 1g	3%
	✓ Sugars 0g	
	✓ Protein 0g	
	✓ Vitamin A	4%
	✓ Vitamin C	6%
	✓ Calcium	2%
	✓ Iron	4%

Instructions:

1. Generously season both sides of chicken with salt and pepper and transfer to a large, re-sealable bag.

2. In a small bowl, whisk together olive oil, lemon juice, garlic, onion powder, lime zest, oregano and red pepper flakes.

3. Pour marinade into plastic bag, seal and move bag around so that chicken is completely coated.

4. Refrigerate chicken for 1-4 hours.

5. When ready, preheat grill (or griddle) to medium-high and cook chicken breasts, flipping in the middle, until no longer pink. 6-8 minutes total.

NOTE: After flipping, drizzle a little of remaining marinade over the top.

Honey Soy Chicken Breast

INGREDIENTS	NUTRITION FACTS (Per Serving)	
1 /4 cup honey	✓ Calories 220	
1/3 cup light soy sauce	✓ Calories from Fat 30	
1/2 tsp ground black pepper (fresh)		
4 cloves minced garlic	**% Daily Value ***	
1 tbsp fresh ginger root (finely grated)	✓ Total Fat 3.5g	5%
4 chicken breasts (large, not boneless, skinless)	✓ Saturated Fat 1g	5%
	✓ Trans Fat	
	✓ Cholesterol 75mg	25%
	✓ Sodium 1330mg	55%
	✓ Potassium 510mg	15%
4 SERVINGS	✓ Total Carbohydrate 20g	7%
TOTAL TIME 70MINS	✓ Dietary Fiber 0g	0%
	✓ Sugars 18g	
	✓ Protein 26g	
	✓ Vitamin A	2%
	✓ Vitamin C	4%
	✓ Calcium	2%
	✓ Iron	4%

Instructions:

1. Stir together all the ingredients except the chicken breasts and pour into a large Ziploc bag.

2. Add the chicken breasts and marinate in the fridge for a couple of hours or overnight.

3.   Place the marinated chicken breasts on an aluminum foil lined cookie sheet and bake at 375 degrees F, uncovered, for about 45 minutes or until the chicken is fully cooked. I use a meat thermometer to make sure the internal temperature is between 170 and 180 degrees F.

4.   Do not throw out the marinade. While the chicken is cooking simmer it over low heat and brush it on the chicken about every 10 minutes as it cooks.

Orange Shrimp

INGREDIENTS	NUTRITION FACTS (Per Serving)	
1 lb medium shrimp (peeled and deveined)	✓ Calories 260	
1/4 tsp ground black pepper (freshly)	✓ Calories from Fat 50	
1/8 cup ketchup	**% Daily Value ***	
1/4 cup orange juice (or blood orange juice)	✓ Total Fat 6g 9%	
	✓ Saturated Fat 0.5g	3%
1/4 cup honey	✓ Trans Fat	
1 tbsp rice vinegar	✓ Cholesterol 175mg	58%
3 cloves garlic (minced)	✓ Sodium 330mg	14%
1/2 tsp red pepper flakes (less or more)	✓ Potassium 360mg	10%
	✓ Total Carbohydrate 26g	9%
1/2 tbsp dried chives (optional)	✓ Dietary Fiber less than 1g	2%
sliced almonds (optional)	✓ Sugars 20g	
chili pepper (Korean wrinkled, sliced, optional)	✓ Protein 26g	
	✓ Vitamin A	8%
1 tbsp corn starch (+ 2 tablespoons water, optional)	✓ Vitamin C	20%
	✓ Calcium	8%
	✓ Iron	15%
4 SERVINGS TOTAL TIME 25MINS		

Instructions:

1. Place shrimp on heated grill (outdoor or indoor). Season them with black pepper and grill until cooked.

2.   To make the sauce: combine soy sauce, ketchup, orange juice, honey, vinegar, garlic, chives (optional), and red pepper flakes in a bowl.

3.   Add the grilled shrimp to a pan over medium high heat. Add the prepared sauce to the pan and stir well. Reduce the heat to low and cook until the sauce thickens, stirring occasionally. (If the sauce does not thicken — Seems to be a problem with a lot of people, then combine cornstarch and water in a small bowl, mix well, then pour it into the sauce, stirring frequently.)

4.   Sprinkle with almonds and Korean wrinkled chili peppers if desired and serve over a bed of steamed white rice.

Tuna Patties

INGREDIENTS	NUTRITION FACTS (Per Serving)		
Salt water	✓	Calories 110	
15 oz. tuna packed in water	✓	Calories from Fat 80	
3 eggs			
2 tbsps lemon juice (about	**% Daily Value ***		
1/2 a large lemon)	✓	Total Fat 9g	14%
1/2 cup purple onion (chopped)	✓	Saturated Fat 1.5g	8%
1 tsp dried parsley	✓	Trans Fat	
1/2 tsp dried dill	✓	Cholesterol 160mg	53%
1 tsp garlic powder	✓	Sodium 55mg	2%
Oil (for cooking)	✓	Potassium 100mg	3%
	✓	Total Carbohydrate 3g	1%
	✓	Dietary Fiber less than 1g	2%
4 SERVINGS (Approximately	✓	Sugars 1g	
12 patties)	✓	Protein 5g	
TOTAL TIME 25MINS	✓	Vitamin A	4%
	✓	Vitamin C	10%
	✓	Calcium	4%
	✓	Iron	6%

Instructions:

1. Stir everything together in a medium-mixing bowl until well combined.

2. Form small patties with your hands (about 1 ½ inches in diameter).

3. Cook in a skillet using heart-healthy oil.

Caprese Meatballs

INGREDIENTS	NUTRITION FACTS	
1 lb ground turkey	✓ Calories 70	
1 eggs	✓ Calories from Fat 40	
1/4 cup almond flour		
1/2 tsp salt	**% Daily Value ***	
1/4 tsp ground black pepper	✓ Total Fat 4.5g	7%
1/2 tsp garlic powder	✓ Saturated Fat 1g	5%
1/2 cup mozzarella cheese	✓ Trans Fat	
(shredded whole milk)	✓ Cholesterol 35mg	12%
2 tbsps sun-dried	✓ Sodium 85mg	4%
tomatoes (chopped)	✓ Potassium 90mg	3%
2 tbsps fresh basil (chopped)	✓ Total Carbohydrate 0g	0%
2 tbsps olive oil (for frying)	✓ Dietary Fiber 0g	0%
	✓ Sugars 0g	
	✓ Protein 6g	
16 MEATBALLS	✓ Vitamin A	2%
TOTAL TIME 30MINS	✓ Vitamin C	0%
	✓ Calcium	2%
	✓ Iron	2%

Instructions:

1. Combine all ingredients except the olive oil in a medium bowl, and mix thoroughly.

2. Form into 16 meatballs.

3. Heat the olive oil in a large nonstick sauté pan. Add the meatballs to the hot oil about 1 inch apart (you may have to do two batches) and cook over low/medium heat for about 3

minutes per side or until cooked through. Because the cheese melts out a bit, be careful that they don't burn - if they appear to be getting dark quickly, then turn down the heat and cook them at a lower temp.

4.   Serve alone, with marinara sauce, or on skewers with fresh mozzarella, basil leaves, and cherry tomatoes. Enjoy!

NOTE: (Approximate nutrition information)

- Per meatball - 78 calories, 6g fat, .5 net carbs, 6g protein

- Per serving (4) - 310 calories, 22g fat, 2g net carbs, 26g protein

Creamy Courgette Lasagna

INGREDIENTS	NUTRITION FACTS (Per Serving)		
9 dried lasagna sheets	✓	Kcalories	405
1 tbsp sunflower oil	✓	Protein	18g
1 onion, finely chopped	✓	Carbs	38g
700g courgettes (about	✓	Fat	21g
6), coarsely grated	✓	Saturates	8g
2 garlic cloves, crushed	✓	Fibre	4g
250g tub ricotta	✓	Sugar	13g
50g cheddar	✓	Salt	1.36g
350g jar tomato sauce for pasta			
4 SERVINGS			
TOTAL TIME 30MINS			

Instructions:

1.   Heat oven to 220C/fan 200C/gas 7.

2.   Put a pan of water on to boil, then cook the lasagna sheets for about 5 mins until softened, but not cooked through. Rinse in cold water, then drizzle with a little oil to stop them sticking together.

3.   Meanwhile, heat the oil in a large frying pan, then fry the onion. After 3 mins, add the courgettes and garlic and continue to fry until the courgette has softened and turned bright green.

4. Stir in 2/3 of both the ricotta and the cheddar, then season to taste. Heat the tomato sauce in the microwave for 2 mins on High until hot.

5. In a large baking dish, layer up the lasagna, starting with half the courgette mix, then pasta, then tomato sauce. Repeat, top with blobs of the remaining ricotta, then scatter with the rest of the cheddar. Bake on the top shelf for about 10 mins until the pasta is tender and the cheese is golden.

Potato, Leek and Feta Tart

INGREDIENTS	NUTRITION FACTS (Per Serving)		
1 tablespoon olive oil	✓	Calories	396
2 leeks (white and light green	✓	Fat	22g
parts), cut into half-moons	✓	Sat Fat	9g
2 small zucchini, cut into half-moons	✓	Cholesterol	27mg
kosher salt and black pepper	✓	Sodium	668mg
1/2 cup crumbled Feta (about 2 ounces)	✓	Protein	7g
2 tablespoons chopped fresh dill	✓	Carbohydrate	44g
2 Red Bliss potatoes (8	✓	Fiber	2g
ounces), thinly sliced			
1 store-bought 9-inch piecrust			
4 SERVINGS			
TOTAL TIME 80MINS			

Instructions:

1.   Heat oven to 375° F.

2.   Heat the oil in a large skillet over medium heat. Add the leeks, zucchini, ½ teaspoon salt, and ¼ teaspoon pepper and cook, stirring occasionally, until just tender, 4 to 5 minutes.

3.   Stir in the Feta and dill. Add the potatoes and toss to combine.

4.   On a piece of parchment paper, roll the piecrust to a 12-inch diameter.

5. Slide the paper onto a baking sheet. Spoon the potato mixture onto the piecrust, leaving a 2-inch border.

6. Fold the edge of the piecrust over the edge of the potato mixture.

7. Bake (covering with foil if the crust gets too dark) until the piecrust is golden brown and the potatoes are tender, 50 to 60 minutes.

Easy Margherita Flatbread Pizza

INGREDIENTS	NUTRITION FACTS (Per Serving)		
1 naan	✓ Calories 240		
3 pieces chees fresh mozzarella (sliced to ⅓- 1/2 inch thickness)	✓ Calories from Fat 120		
1 tomatoes (sliced as thin as possible)	**% Daily Value ***		
	✓ Total Fat 13g	20%	
6 leaves basil	✓ Saturated Fat 2g	10%	
3 cloves garlic (pressed; or 1 tsp dry garlic powder)	✓ Trans Fat		
	✓ Cholesterol 0%		
11/2 tbsps olive oil	✓ Sodium 620mg	26%	
11/2 tbsps balsamic vinegar	✓ Potassium 300mg	9%	
Salt	✓ Total Carbohydrate 27g		9%
Pepper	✓ Dietary Fiber 3g	12%	
	✓ Sugars 4g		
2 SERVINGS	✓ Protein 4g		
TOTAL TIME 15MINS	✓ Vitamin A 10%		
	✓ Vitamin C 20%		
	✓ Calcium 10%		
	✓ Iron 15%		

Instructions:

1. Press fresh garlic and mix with oil.

2. Brush the flatbread with oil & garlic with half the mixture. Place in preheated to 350F oven for 5 minutes to crisp up.

3. Remove from oven and place 3 slices of cheese on top of the flatbread, sprinkle with salt & pepper, then place thinly sliced tomatoes on top and repeat with a sprinkling of salt & pepper.

Place back in the oven for another 5 minutes, plus extra 2-3 minutes on broil. Watch the bread closely, if it's too dark before 2-3 minutes remove it from the oven immediately.

4. Meanwhile mix the remaining oil & garlic with the balsamic vinegar, stirring until a smooth emulsion forms.

5. Chop the basil leaves.

6. Once flatbread pizza is baked and the edges are golden in color, remove from the oven, drizzle with however much of the balsamic vinegar mixture you would like, sprinkle with basil leaves, slice and serve and enjoy!

Vegetarian Chili

INGREDIENTS	NUTRITION FACTS (Per Serving)
1 tbsp olive oil	Calories 113
2 cups sweet onion (diced, approx. ¾ of a large Vidalia)	Calories from Fat 20
1 poblano peppers (cut into batons, narrow 1 inch strips)	**% Daily Value ***
	Total Fat 2g 3%
2 cloves garlic (minced)	Saturated Fat 0g 0%
1 zucchini (small, diced)	Trans Fat
1 yellow summer squash (small, diced)	Cholesterol 0%
2 tbsps chili powder	Sodium 670mg 28%
1 tsp kosher salt	Potassium 410mg 12%
1 tsp cumin	Total Carbohydrate 12g 4%
1 tsp oregano	Dietary Fiber 4g 16%
1 tsp cilantro	Sugars 6g
1/2 tsp smoked paprika	Protein 2g
1/4 tsp cayenne	Vitamin A 190%
1/4 tsp white pepper	Vitamin C 30%
2 bay leaves	Calcium 6%
15 oz. pumpkin purée (Libby's)	Iron 8%
15 oz. diced tomatoes (with chilies or without)	
15 oz. low sodium black beans (drained and rinsed)	
2 tbsps pickled jalapenos (chopped)	
3 cups vegetable stock (chicken or beef is fine if you are not vegetarian)	
8 SERVINGS	
TOTAL TIME 90MINS	

Instructions:

1. Place Dutch oven or stockpot over med-high heat, add oil, once hot add the onion, Poblano and garlic, sauté 5 minutes, then add the zucchini and yellow squash and sauté another 5 minutes.

2. Add the salt and spices, stir for 1 minute, then add the remaining ingredients. Stir. As soon as the pot starts to bubble, reduce to simmer and cover, to simmer for 1 hour.

3. Serve hot.

4. Garnish with chopped scallions, fresh cilantro or chives. If you are not vegan, a dollop of rich sour cream makes a nice topping.

Stuffed with Mushrooms

INGREDIENTS	NUTRITION FACTS (Per Serving)		
Cabbage - 8-10 leaves	✓	Calories 90	
Water	✓	Calories from Fat 60	
Vegetable oil - 2 tbsp			
For the filling:	**% Daily Value ***		
Fresh mushrooms - 500 g or	✓	Total Fat 7g	11%
dried mushrooms - 100 g	✓	Saturated Fat 0g	0%
Tomato paste - 1-2 tbsp. l.	✓	Trans Fat 0g	
Loose rice porridge - 1/2 Art.	✓	Cholesterol	0%
Salt - to taste	✓	Sodium 450mg	19%
	✓	Potassium 85mg	2%
4 SERVINGS	✓	Total Carbohydrate 6g 2%	
TOTAL TIME 50MINS	✓	Dietary Fiber 0g	0%
	✓	Sugars less than 1g	
	✓	Protein less than 1g	
	✓	Vitamin A	2%
	✓	Vitamin C	4%
	✓	Calcium	0%
	✓	Iron	2%

Instructions:

1. Boil the cabbage leaves in boiling water for 2-3 min., Removed from the water, let the water drain out.

2. If necessary, hard veins of the leaves lightly beat off until soft wooden hoe.

3.   For each cabbage leaf to put 2-3 tablespoons of filling and wrap it. Stuffed cabbage fry in oil, then stew or baking dish in the oven on a baking sheet.

4.   Serve with boiled potatoes and cucumber salad.

5.   For the filling wash the dried mushrooms and boil, boil fresh mushrooms, finely chopped, mixed with rice and tomato paste, salt to taste.

Sugar Free, Guilt Free Recipes

The idea of eliminating sugar in our diet is resetting our insulin and you know how important the role of insulin is in weight gain/weight loss. We're also going to eliminate our sugar cravings through this diet.

Spaetzle

INGREDIENTS	NUTRITION FACTS (Per Serving)
⅔ cups (80 grams) white all-purpose, unbleached flour ⅓ cup (40 grams) whole wheat flour 2 tsp. kosher salt, divided ¼ tsp. fresh ground black pepper Pinch of nutmeg ½ cup egg substitute or equivalent of 2 eggs ¼ cup 2% fat milk 4 SERVINGS TOTAL TIME 75MINS	Calories 140 Calories from Fat 15 **% Daily Value *** Total Fat 1.5g 2% Saturated Fat 0g 0% Trans Fat Cholesterol less than 5 mg 1% Sodium 690mg 29% Potassium 190mg 5% Total Carbohydrate 24g 8% Dietary Fiber 2g 8% Sugars 1g Protein 8g Vitamin A 0% Vitamin C 0% Calcium 4% Iron 10%

Instructions:

1. In a large bowl, mix both flour, 1 tsp. kosher salt, pepper and nutmeg.

2. Make a well in the middle and add egg substitute and milk.

3. Stir until batter is smooth.

4. Bring a large pot of water to boil. Add 1 tsp. kosher salt.

5.   Pour batter into a spaetzle maker or colander placed over the pot of boiling water. Push the batter slowly through. Use a spatula to push the batter through if you are using a colander.

6.   Stir the spaetzle frequently. It should be floating. Cook for another 2 minutes.

Sweet Potato Fries

INGREDIENTS	NUTRITION FACTS (Per Serving)		
2 sweet potatoes (sliced into 1/2" thick wedges)	Calories 90		
1 tbsp olive oil	Calories from Fat 30		
kosher salt (to taste)			
ground black pepper (freshly, to taste)	**% Daily Value ***		
garlic powder (to taste)	Total Fat 3.5g	5%	
	Saturated Fat 0g	0%	
	Trans Fat		
4 SERVINGS	Cholesterol	0%	
TOTAL TIME 40MINS	Sodium 230mg	10%	
	Potassium 250mg	7%	
	Total Carbohydrate 15g		5%
	Dietary Fiber 2g	8%	
	Sugars 3g		
	Protein 2g		
	Vitamin A		180%
	Vitamin C	2%	
	Calcium 2%		
	Iron	6%	

Instructions:

1. Preheat oven to 425 degrees F. Line a baking sheet with foil. If you are using regular foil be sure to spray it well with cooking spray.

2. Place sweet potato wedges in a bowl and add 1 tablespoon olive oil (more or less as needed to coat the fries), 1-2

teaspoons salt to taste, 1/2 - 1 teaspoon fresh black pepper to taste, and 1-2 teaspoons garlic powder to taste.

NOTE: Because sweet potatoes vary in size, the amount of seasoning you use will vary. Use more or less as needed. The more you make this recipe the easier it will be to 'guess' what is right for you. Toss the potatoes to coat them evenly with oil and seasonings and place them on the prepared baking sheet.

3.   Be sure the sweet potato wedges are in one layer and there is space around each wedge. Leaving space around each potato wedge is important for getting them a little crispy. If they are crowded they will steam and be soggy.

4.   Bake the sweet potato fries for about 15 minutes and then turn each fry over and bake another 10-15 minutes. Watch them carefully so they don't burn. Keep in mind the cook time will vary depending on the size of your fries. If they are thick like steak fries you will need to cook them longer. If they are thin you will want to shorten the cook time.

Skinny Bang Bang Cauliflower

INGREDIENTS	NUTRITION FACTS (Per Serving)		
1/2 head cauliflower (cut into bite sized florets)	✓ Calories 320		
	✓ Calories from Fat 70		
11/2 cups panko breadcrumbs (Kikkoman brand preferred for even baking)	**% Daily Value ***		
2 large eggs (whisked)	✓ Total Fat 7g 11%		
1 tbsp fresh parsley (finely chopped, optional, for garnish)	✓ Saturated Fat 2g	10%	
	✓ Trans Fat		
2 tbsps sweet chili sauce (I bought mine from an Asian grocery store. Make sure to buy the kind that is a smooth sauce without chili seeds)	✓ Cholesterol 280mg	93%	
	✓ Sodium 660mg	28%	
	✓ Potassium 790mg	23%	
	✓ Total Carbohydrate		
2 tsps hot sauce (I used sriracha)	51g 17%		
1/4 cup greek style plain yogurt (fat free, try to use a thicker consistency one like Fage)	✓ Dietary Fiber 5g	20%	
	✓ Sugars 21g		
1 tbsp honey	✓ Protein 16g		
	✓ Vitamin A 15%		
2 SERVINGS	✓ Vitamin C 180%		
TOTAL TIME 40MINS	✓ Calcium 10%		
	✓ Iron 10%		

Instructions:

1. Preheat oven to 400F. Dip cauliflower pieces in egg and then roll in panko until fully coated and place on a baking sheet lined with parchment paper. You will need to use your fingers to press on the coating to help it to stick to the cauliflower bites. Repeat until all cauliflower is coated.

2. Bake for about 20 minutes or until coating is a dark golden brown and crunchy.

3. While cauliflower is cooking, make the bang bang sauce. Add all ingredients into a small bowl and whisk until uniform and no yogurt lumps remain (a whisk is a better tool to get the yogurt lumps out than a fork). Drizzle over finished cauliflower, reserving additional for dipping. Garnish with fresh parsley if desired.

Healthy Garlic Mashed Potatoes

INGREDIENTS	NUTRITION FACTS (Per Serving)		
2 lbs russet potatoes	✓ Calories 320		
1/2 lb cauliflower	✓ Calories from Fat 110		
4 tbsps butter			
6 cloves garlic (minced)	**% Daily Value ***		
1/2 cup chicken broth	✓ Total Fat 12g	18%	
1/2 cup skim milk	✓ Saturated Fat 7g	35%	
sea salt (to taste)	✓ Trans Fat		
	✓ Cholesterol 30mg	10%	
4 SERVINGS	✓ Sodium 330mg	14%	
TOTAL TIME 45MINS	✓ Potassium 1210mg	35%	
	✓ Total Carbohydrate 47g		16%
	✓ Dietary Fiber 3g	12%	
	✓ Sugars 5g		
	✓ Protein 8g		
	✓ Vitamin A 10%		
	✓ Vitamin C 70%		
	✓ Calcium 10%		
	✓ Iron 15%		

Instructions:

1. Peel potatoes, leaving a little bit of the skin on here and there. Wash the potatoes thoroughly and cut into large chunks. Place the prepped potatoes in a large pot.

2. Wash the cauliflower and break into large chunks. Add to the pot and cover the potatoes and cauliflower with water. Bring

to a boil over high heat, then reduce heat to maintain a gentle boil. Cook until the potatoes fall apart when poked.

3.   Drain the potatoes and cauliflower and set aside temporarily. Rinse the pot out well and return it to the stove over medium high heat.

4.   Add the butter and garlic to the pot and salute until the garlic is golden brown. Reduce the heat to low and return the potatoes and cauliflower to the pot. Add the broth and milk. Mash/mis using a potato masher for a chunkier mashed potato and a spoon or use an immersion blender to produce creamy potatoes. Add sea salt to taste and stir well. Serve hot.

Skinny Chocolate Cheesecake

INGREDIENTS	NUTRITION FACTS (Per Serving)		
1/2 cup walnuts (finely ground)	✓ Calories 120		
1 tbsp coconut oil	✓ Calories from Fat 70		
1 tsp honey			
16 oz. low-fat cream cheese	**% Daily Value ***		
1 cup greek yogurt (vanilla)	✓ Total Fat 8g 12%		
1/4 cup honey	✓ Saturated Fat 4g	20%	
3 tbsps cocoa powder	✓ Trans Fat		
1 tbsp vanilla extract	✓ Cholesterol 15mg	5%	
1/4 tsp sea salt	✓ Sodium 160mg	7%	
	✓ Potassium 130mg	4%	
16 SERVINGS	✓ Total Carbohydrate 9g 3%		
TOTAL TIME 30MINS	✓ Dietary Fiber less than 1g		2%
	✓ Sugars 7g		
	✓ Protein 4g		
	✓ Vitamin A 4%		
	✓ Vitamin C 0%		
	✓ Calcium 8%		
	✓ Iron 2%		

Instructions:

1. Combine the crust ingredients in a bowl and press into a square baking dish.

2. Put the cheesecake ingredients in a food processor and puree until smooth and creamy. Spread the mixture into the baking dish and refrigerate for at least 3 hours.

3. Cut into squares and serve.

Breakfast Sticks

INGREDIENTS	NUTRITION FACTS (Per Serving)	
1 tbsp oil (choice)	✓ Calories 70	
2 slices bacon (chopped)	✓ Calories from Fat 60	
3 oz. breakfast sausages		
2 green onions (large, chopped)	**% Daily Value ***	
4 large eggs (beaten)	✓ Total Fat 6g	9%
1 oz jack cheese	✓ Saturated Fat 2g	10%
(shredded Monterrey)	✓ Trans Fat	
	✓ Cholesterol 110mg	37%
8 SERVINGS	✓ Sodium 70mg	3%
TOTAL TIME 35MINS	✓ Potassium 50mg	1%
	✓ Total Carbohydrate less than 1g	0%
	✓ Dietary Fiber 0g	0%
	✓ Sugars 0g	
	✓ Protein 4g	
	✓ Vitamin A	4%
	✓ Vitamin C	2%
	✓ Calcium	4%
	✓ Iron	4%

Instructions:

1.   Preheat oven to 350º. Oil your muffin/pan slots with oil using a brush and set aside.

2.   Beat the eggs with the shredded cheese in a medium mixing bowl and set aside. Using a non-stick skillet, brown the bacon.

3.   Add the sausage crumbled, stirring and cooking until it is no longer pink.

4.   Add onion and sauté just until onion begins to cook/wilt. Remove from heat and cool 1-2 minutes.

5.   Add the meat mixture to the egg mixture and beat together well with a spoon. Using a ¼c. measuring cup, scoop up ¼ c. of the mixture into each of 8 slots.

6.   Pop into preheated 350° oven for about 15-20 minutes (ovens do vary) until just set and barely beginning to brown on tops. Remove from pans/slot with a knife tip and serve at once.

Seared Scallops with Asparagus Sauce

INGREDIENTS	NUTRITION FACTS (Per Serving)	
6 sea scallops	✓ Calories 370	
salt	✓ Calories from Fat 290	
1 lb asparagus		
1/2 cup chicken broth	**% Daily Value ***	
(warm, if cooking gluten-	✓ Total Fat 32g	49%
free use gluten-free stock)	✓ Saturated Fat 12g	60%
3 tbsps butter	✓ Trans Fat	
2 tbsps canola oil (or other	✓ Cholesterol 60mg	20%
high smoke-point oil)	✓ Sodium 610mg	25%
	✓ Potassium 660mg	19%
2 SERVINGS	✓ Total Carbohydrate 11g	4%
TOTAL TIME 40MINS	✓ Dietary Fiber 5g	20%
	✓ Sugars 5g	
	✓ Protein 14g	
	✓ Vitamin A 45%	
	✓ Vitamin C 25%	
	✓ Calcium 8%	
	✓ Iron 25%	

Instructions:

1. Salt the scallops well and set aside at room temperature while you make the asparagus sauce.

2. Steam the asparagus for the sauce. Use a potato peeler to shave the outer layer off the asparagus spears, up to about three-quarters of the way up the spear. This part is more fibrous and will not break down as well in the blender. Chop

into 2-inch pieces. Boil the asparagus in a pot of salted water for 5-8 minutes. This is longer than you'd normally cook asparagus, but you want the spears to blend well later.

3. Remove the asparagus from the pot. If you want to retain that vibrant green color, shock them in an ice bath. Put them in a food processor or blender. Add half the chicken stock and purée until smooth. (If you want an even smoother texture you can push the purée through a fine mesh sieve or a food mill.) Pour the sauce into a small pot and add the butter. Heat over very low heat until the butter melts, but do not let it boil, or even simmer. The sauce should be warm, not hot. If the sauce is too thick you can add more chicken stock. Add salt to taste.

4. Pat the scallops dry with a paper towel. Heat a sauté pan on high heat. Add a high smoke point oil like canola or grape seed oil, and let it heat up for 2 minutes. The pan should be very hot. If it starts to smoke, move the pan off the heat. Lay in the scallops in the pan, well separated from each other. You might need to sear in batches.

5. If your scallops are thicker than 1 inch, turn the heat down to medium-high. Most sea scallops are about an inch. Let them sear without moving for at least 3-4 minutes. Keep an eye on them. You will see a crust beginning to form on the

outside edge of the scallop, and the meat will begin to whiten upward. A good time to check the scallop is when you see a golden brown ring at the edge of the scallop. Try picking it up with tongs, and if it comes cleanly, check it – you should see a deep golden sear. If not, let it back down and keep searing.

6. When the scallops are well seared on one side, turn them over and sear on high heat for 1 minute (give or take). Then turn off the heat. The residual heat will continue to cook the scallops for a few minutes. Let the scallops cook for at least another minute, or more if you like your scallops well done.

7. To serve pour a little sauce in the middle of the plate, top with the scallops, the more browned side up.

8. Serve at once. Garnish with a little chopped parsley if you want, and maybe with a wedge of lemon.

Raspberry and Banana Smoothie

INGREDIENTS	NUTRITION FACTS (Per Serving)		
2/3 cup yoghurt natural low fat	✓ Calories 120		
1 cup low-fat milk	✓ Calories from Fat 15		
1 cup frozen raspberries			
1 bananas	**% Daily Value ***		
1 tbsp bran (natural)	✓ Total Fat 2g 3%		
1 tbsp honey	✓ Saturated Fat 1g	5%	
	✓ Trans Fat		
4 SERVINGS	✓ Cholesterol less than 5 mg		2%
TOTAL TIME 15MINS	✓ Sodium 55mg	2%	
	✓ Potassium 360mg	10%	
	✓ Total Carbohydrate 22g		7%
	✓ Dietary Fiber 4g	16%	
	✓ Sugars 15g		
	✓ Protein 5g		
	✓ Vitamin A 4%		
	✓ Vitamin C 20%		
	✓ Calcium 15%		
	✓ Iron 4%		

Instructions:

1. Place all ingredients into a blender and mix until smooth.

2. Place into 2 glasses and serve immediately.

Raspberry and Banana Pancakes

INGREDIENTS	NUTRITION FACTS (Per Serving)		
1 cup self rising flour	✓ Calories 250		
1 eggs	✓ Calories from Fat 40		
1 cup milk			
1/2 tsp vanilla	**% Daily Value ***		
1 cup yoghurt natural low fat	✓ Total Fat 4.5g	7%	
2 tsps powdered sugar (or honey)	✓ Saturated Fat 1.5g	8%	
1 cup frozen raspberries	✓ Trans Fat		
(defrosted)	✓ Cholesterol 60mg	20%	
1 bananas (sliced)	✓ Sodium 490mg	20%	
cooking spray	✓ Potassium 470mg	13%	
	✓ Total Carbohydrate 43g		14%
4 SERVINGS	✓ Dietary Fiber 5g	20%	
TOTAL TIME 30MINS	✓ Sugars 14g		
	✓ Protein 11g		
	✓ Vitamin A 4%		
	✓ Vitamin C 25%		
	✓ Calcium 30%		
	✓ Iron 10%		

Instructions:

1. In a large mixing bowl, sift flour and make a well in the centre. Crack egg into centre and pour the milk on top with vanilla essence. Wisk until smooth. Place in fridge for 30 mins.

2. Once raspberries have thawed gently mix them with the yoghurt, sugar and set aside.

3. Heat a non-stick frying pan on med heat with a spray of cooking spray. Pour some of the pancake mixture into the centre of the pan. When it starts bubbling around the edges it is ready to flip over. If making large pancakes it will take around 4 mins each side.

4. Place on plate when ready, divide the yoghurt mixture on top, slice banana and enjoy!

Raspberry and Banana Pancakes

INGREDIENTS	NUTRITION FACTS (Per Serving)		
1 cup self rising flour	✓ Calories 250		
5 oz. arugula (organic, pre-washed)	✓ Calories from Fat 40		
1/2 pt strawberries (organic, washed and sliced)	**% Daily Value ***		
2 oz. soft goat's cheese (crumbled)	✓ Total Fat 4.5g	7%	
2 tbsps nuts (your choice)	✓ Saturated Fat 1.5g	8%	
pepper	✓ Trans Fat		
salt	✓ Cholesterol 60mg	20%	
vinaigrette (Lemon, to taste)	✓ Sodium 490mg	20%	
	✓ Potassium 470mg	13%	
4 SERVINGS	✓ Total Carbohydrate 43g		14%
TOTAL TIME 5MINS	✓ Dietary Fiber 5g	20%	
	✓ Sugars 14g		
	✓ Protein 11g		
	✓ Vitamin A	4%	
	✓ Vitamin C	25%	
	✓ Calcium	30%	
	✓ Iron	10%	

Instructions:

1. Place greens in a large bowl.

2. Top with remaining ingredients and a tiny pinch of salt & pepper.

3. Drizzle with desired amount of dressing and toss before serving.

Fruitless and Loving it Recipes

In this section, we're eliminating fruits. Fruits may be food items that are considered healthy but eliminating it will reset the hunger hormone leptin.

Tuna Salad

INGREDIENTS	NUTRITION FACTS (Per Serving)		
1 can albacore	✓ Calories 190		
2/3 cup nonfat cottage cheese	✓ Calories from Fat 0		
4 tbsps low-fat plain yogurt			
1/4 purple onion (small, chopped finely)	**% Daily Value ***		
	✓ Total Fat 0g 0%		
1 stalk celery (chopped finely)	✓ Saturated Fat 0g	0%	
1 tsp Dijon mustard	✓ Trans Fat		
lemon juice (splash of)	✓ Cholesterol less than 5 mg		1%
2 dill	✓ Sodium 95mg	4%	
	✓ Potassium 90mg	3%	
	✓ Total Carbohydrate 4g 1%		
2 SERVINGS	✓ Dietary Fiber 0g	0%	
TOTAL TIME 12MINS	✓ Sugars 2g		
	✓ Protein 3g		
	✓ Vitamin A 2%		
	✓ Vitamin C 6%		
	✓ Calcium 6%		
	✓ Iron 0%		

Instructions:

1. Just throw into a bowl, give it a good mix and ENJOY!

Breakfast Burrito Bites

INGREDIENTS	NUTRITION FACTS (Per Serving)	
3 tbsps chopped bell pepper	✓ Calories 100	
1 tsp olive oil (or spray pan with non stick cooking spray)	✓ Calories from Fat 50	
3 eggs (whipped slightly in a bowl)	**% Daily Value ***	
1 tbsp water	✓ Total Fat 6g 9%	
2 whole whole wheat tortillas	✓ Saturated Fat 1.5g	8%
	✓ Trans Fat	
4 SERVINGS	✓ Cholesterol 160mg	53%
TOTAL TIME 20MINS	✓ Sodium 130mg	5%
	✓ Potassium 70mg	2%
	✓ Total Carbohydrate 6g 2%	
	✓ Dietary Fiber 0g	0%
	✓ Sugars less than 1g	
	✓ Protein 6g	
	✓ Vitamin A 4%	
	✓ Vitamin C 0%	
	✓ Calcium 4%	
	✓ Iron 6%	

Instructions:

1. Cook peppers with oil or cooking spray.

2. Remove peppers from pan.

3. Whisk eggs and water together. Cook egg/water mixture over hot skillet, without scrambling them.

4. Move egg inward to cook although through, and flip, so you have a large "fried egg". Cut in half. Place one egg on each tortilla.

5. Add peppers to the center of your tortilla and roll up.

Meatloaf for Dinner

INGREDIENTS	NUTRITION FACTS (Per Serving)	
3/4 cup onions (diced)	✓ Calories 260	
2 lbs ground meat (meat loaf mix, ground pork, beef and veal)	✓ Calories from Fat 120	
1/2 cup ketchup	**% Daily Value ***	
1/2 cup mustard (Dijon adds a nice bite)	✓ Total Fat 13g	20%
2 eggs (beaten)	✓ Saturated Fat 5g	25%
1 cup bread crumbs (seasoned)	✓ Trans Fat 1g	
salt (and pepper, to taste *)	✓ Cholesterol 125mg	42%
	✓ Sodium 570mg	24%
	✓ Potassium 490mg	14%
8 SERVINGS	✓ Total Carbohydrate 9g 3%	
TOTAL TIME 105MINS	✓ Dietary Fiber less than 1g	4%
	✓ Sugars 5g	
	✓ Protein 26g	
	✓ Vitamin A 4%	
	✓ Vitamin C 6%	
	✓ Calcium 4%	
	✓ Iron 20%	

Instructions:

1. Preheat the oven to 350 degrees.

2. In a large mixing bowl, combine all ingredients and mix until evenly combined. Mix it up with your hands, get a little dirty, it's all good.

3. When we salt and pepper says to taste in this case, we do not mean you should taste this raw meat mixture. That instruction just means add as much salt and pepper as you'd like. A good sprinkle of each should do it.

4. You can make one large loaf or two small loafs from your mixture. Either way place your loaf/ loaves onto a baking sheet. Place in the preheated oven for 1 hour for 1 large loaf. If you are going for 2 smaller loaves, reduce cooking time to about 45 minutes.

5. For an easy glaze you can top the loaf/ loaves with barbecue sauce or ketchup half way through cooking.

Cauliflower Tortillas

INGREDIENTS	NUTRITION FACTS (Per Serving)	
¾ head cauliflower	✓ Calories 50	
2 large eggs	✓ Calories from Fat 15	
¼ cup chopped cilantro fresh		
½ lime (add the zest too if you	**% Daily Value ***	
want more of a lime flavor)	✓ Total Fat 1.5g	2%
Salt & pepper	✓ Saturated Fat 0.5g	3%
	✓ Trans Fat	
	✓ Cholesterol 70mg	23%
6 SERVINGS	✓ Sodium 180mg	8%
TOTAL TIME 50MINS	✓ Potassium 280mg	8%
	✓ Total Carbohydrate 6g	2%
	✓ Dietary Fiber 2g	8%
	✓ Sugars 2g	
	✓ Protein 4g	
	✓ Vitamin A	4%
	✓ Vitamin C	60%
	✓ Calcium	4%
	✓ Iron	6%

Instructions:

1. Preheat the oven to 375 degrees F. and line a baking sheet with parchment paper.

2. Trim the cauliflower, cut it into small, uniform pieces, and pulse in a food processor in batches until you get a couscous-like consistency. The finely riced cauliflower should make about 2 cups packed.

3. Place the cauliflower in a microwave-safe bowl and microwave for 2 minutes, then stir and microwave again for another 2 minutes. Place the cauliflower in a fine cheesecloth or thin dishtowel and squeeze out as much liquid as possible, being careful not to burn yourself. Dishwashing gloves are suggested as it is very hot.

4. In a medium bowl, whisk the eggs. Add in cauliflower, cilantro, lime, salt and pepper. Mix until well combined. Use your hands to shape 6 small "tortillas" on the parchment paper.

5. Bake for 10 minutes, carefully flip each tortilla, and return to the oven for an additional 5 to 7 minutes, or until completely set. Place tortillas on a wire rack to cool slightly.

6. Heat a medium-sized skillet on medium. Place a baked tortilla in the pan, pressing down slightly, and brown for 1 to 2 minutes on each side. Repeat with remaining tortillas.

TIP: You can munch on these by themselves, make quesadillas with them, or add some taco filling and fold it like a taco.

Baked Herb Salmon

INGREDIENTS	NUTRITION FACTS (Per Serving)	
4 salmon fillets (thawed according to packaging)	✓ Calories 240	
1 tsp dill weed	✓ Calories from Fat 130	
1 tsp dried rosemary	**% Daily Value ***	
1/2 tsp parsley	✓ Total Fat 15g	23%
1/2 tsp salt	✓ Saturated Fat 3.5g	18%
1/4 tsp pepper	✓ Trans Fat	
	✓ Cholesterol 60mg	20%
4 SERVINGS	✓ Sodium 360mg	15%
TOTAL TIME 25MINS	✓ Potassium 450mg	13%
	✓ Total Carbohydrate 3g	1%
	✓ Dietary Fiber 1g	4%
	✓ Sugars 0g	
	✓ Protein 23g	
	✓ Vitamin A	2%
	✓ Vitamin C	40%
	✓ Calcium	4%
	✓ Iron	2%

Instructions:

1. Preheat over to 400 degrees. Prepare cookie sheet by linking with parchment paper or aluminum foil.

2. Mix dill weed, rosemary, parsley, salt and pepper together in a little bowl.

3. Place salmon on cookie sheet.

4. Sprinkle each salmon with herbs.

5.   Bake for 20 minutes or until internal temperature of the salmon reaches 145 degrees.

6.   Serve with favorite sides.

Quinoa "Fried Rice"

INGREDIENTS	NUTRITION FACTS (Per Serving)		
1 tbsp olive oil (divided)	✓ Calories 210		
2 fried eggs (large, chopped, pre-cook these)	✓ Calories from Fat 35		
2 cloves garlic (minced)	**% Daily Value ***		
1 onions (small, diced)	✓ Total Fat 4g 6%		
8 oz. mushrooms (chopped)	✓ Saturated Fat 0g	0%	
1 head broccoli (or 10oz frozen broccoli, chopped)	✓ Trans Fat		
1 zucchini (chopped)	✓ Cholesterol 0%		
1/2 cup frozen corn	✓ Sodium 510mg	21%	
1/2 cup frozen peas	✓ Potassium 800mg	23%	
1/2 cup carrots (grated)	✓ Total Carbohydrate 34g		11%
3 cups cooked quinoa	✓ Dietary Fiber 8g	32%	
1 tbsp ginger (grated)	✓ Sugars 6g		
3 tbsps soy sauce	✓ Protein 10g		
2 green onions (chopped)	✓ Vitamin A 50%		
	✓ Vitamin C 170%		
6 SERVINGS	✓ Calcium 10%		
TOTAL TIME 40MINS	✓ Iron 15%		

Instructions:

1. Heat 1 TBS olive oil in a large skillet over medium high heat. Add garlic, ginger, and onion and cook for a few minutes until tender.

2. Add mushrooms, broccoli, carrots, and zucchini. Cook for a few more minutes until veggies are tender, stirring often.

3. Add corn, peas, and quinoa. Cook a few more minutes, mixing to distribute heat, until everything is completely heated.

4. Add soy sauce and stir to combine. Then add green onions and eggs, and mix until combined.

5. Serve and garnish with additional green onions.

Zucchini Chips

INGREDIENTS	NUTRITION FACTS (Per Serving)		
1 (large) zucchini, cut into 1/8" - 1/4" slices	✓	Calories	99
1/3 cup whole grain breadcrumbs, optional Panko (homemade breadcrumb recipe)	✓	Total Fat	3g
	✓	Saturated Fat	2g
	✓	Trans Fat	0g
	✓	Cholesterol	13
1/4 cup finely grated parmesan cheese, reduced fat	✓	Carbohydrates	12g
	✓	Sodium	241mg
1/4 teaspoon black pepper	✓	Dietary Fiber	2g
Kosher or sea salt to taste	✓	Sugars	2g
1/8 teaspoon garlic powder	✓	Protein	6g
1/8 teaspoon cayenne pepper			
3 tablespoons low-fat milk			
4 SERVINGS TOTAL TIME 60MINS			

Instructions:

1. Preheat oven to 425 degrees.

2. Combine in a small mixing bowl, breadcrumbs, Parmesan cheese, black pepper, salt, garlic powder, and cayenne pepper.

3. Dip zucchini slices into milk and dredge into bread crumbs to coat both sides.

NOTE: It may be necessary to press crumbs onto zucchini slices to ensure the crumbs stick.

4.   Arrange zucchini on a non-stick cookie sheet and lightly mist with a non-stick cooking spray.

5.   Or, place zucchini on a wire rack sprayed with non-stick cooking spray. If using a rack, place rack on a cookie sheet.

6.   Bake 15 minutes, turn over and continue baking until golden, approximately 10-15 minutes (being careful not to burn).

7.   Allow to cool to room temperature before storing in an airtight container.

NOTE: Zucchini Chips will continue to get crispier while cooling. For gluten free chips, use gluten-free bread crumbs.

Savory French Toast BLT

INGREDIENTS
✓   8 slices bacon
✓   4 large eggs, lightly beaten
✓   3/4 cup heavy cream
✓   1/4 cup chopped fresh chives, plus more for serving
✓   Coarse salt and ground pepper
✓   3 tablespoons unsalted butter
✓   4 slices crusty bread, cut 1 inch thick
✓   4 lettuce leaves (romaine, Boston, or Bibb)
4 SERVINGS
TOTAL TIME 30MINS

Instructions:

1. Preheat oven to 375. Place bacon on a rimmed baking sheet; cook until golden and crisp, about 15 minutes, rotating sheet halfway through. Drain on paper towels.

2. Meanwhile, in a large shallow dish, whisk together eggs, cream, and chives; season with salt and pepper. Lay bread in a single layer in egg mixture and soak 3 minutes on each side. In a large skillet, melt butter over medium. When butter sizzles, add bread and cook until golden and crisp around edges, about 3 minutes per side, flipping once.

3. To serve, layer lettuce, tomato, and bacon on each slice French toast and sprinkle with chives.

Portabella and Halloumi "Burgers"

INGREDIENTS	NUTRITION FACTS (Per Serving)	
7 oz. beef fillet	✓ Calories 310	
7 oz. chicken breasts	✓ Calories from Fat 160	
7 oz. pork tenderloin		
Marinade (Beef)	**% Daily Value ***	
1 tbsp balsamic vinegar	✓ Total Fat 17g	26%
1/2 tbsp olive oil	✓ Saturated Fat 5g	25%
Pepper and salt	✓ Trans Fat	
Marinade (Chicken)	✓ Cholesterol 100mg	33%
1/2 tbsp tarragon	✓ Sodium 530mg	22%
2 cloves garlic (crushed)	✓ Potassium 650mg	19%
1/2 tbsp olive oil	✓ Total Carbohydrate 7g	2%
Marinade (Pork Tenderloin)	✓ Dietary Fiber 2g	8%
2 tbsps sauce (Hoi Sin)	✓ Sugars 2g	
1 tsp sesame oil	✓ Protein 31g	
1/2 tsp ginger (Finely Chopped)	✓ Vitamin A 2%	
	✓ Vitamin C 10%	
	✓ Calcium 6%	
4 SERVINGS	✓ Iron 15%	
TOTAL TIME 20MINS		

Instructions:

1. Cube all the meat so they are roughly the same size. I made approximately 1 1/2 inch cubes of each and got 9 cubes from each of the beef, pork and chicken.

NOTE: If you like your beef medium rare, please cut the chicken a little smaller so it cooks faster than the beef, or put the chicken on a separate skewer so it has more time to cook.

2. Place the pork, beef and chicken in to 3 separate bowls and add the marinade ingredients relating to each meat. Combine the marinade well.

3. Using metal skewers if you have (the heat will conduct better through the meat), start by pushing a piece of beef, then pork, then chicken, and repeat, so you have 2 or 3 cubes of chicken, beef and pork on each skewer. Place on a tray and cover and refrigerate for 20 minutes then BBQ when you are ready!

Portabella and Halloumi "Burgers"

INGREDIENTS
✓ 4 portabella mushroom caps with stems removed
✓ 3 ½ tablespoons balsamic vinegar
✓ 2 tablespoons olive oil
✓ 2 thin slices halloumi
✓ Sea salt and pepper
✓ 1 handful basil leaves
2 SERVINGS
TOTAL TIME 15MINS

Instructions:

1. Heat grill to medium-high heat (about 450 degrees).

2. Wash mushroom caps and cry.

3. In a shallow bowl, combine the balsamic vinegar and olive oil. Place mushrooms gill side down in the mixture.

4. When the grill is hot, grill the mushrooms on the gill side first for about 5 minutes or until they start to sweat. Flip and grill 2-3 minutes more.

5. Add halloumi to the grill and grill 2 minutes on each side over relatively high heat until grill marks form on the cheese and it becomes soft and pliable.

6. Assemble the "burger" with the mushroom as the bun, the halloumi cheese as the burger, the lightly salted tomato and fresh basil leaves.

7. Wrap and serve hot.

Ban the Caffeine Recipes

Banning caffeine will reset your stress and your hormone cortisol.

Soothing Tea Latte

INGREDIENTS	NUTRITION FACTS (Per Serving)		
1 cup boiling water	✓ Calories 60		
1 Tbsp. sugar	✓ Calories from Fat 0		
1/2 cup soy or 2% milk			
1 cinnamon stick	**% Daily Value ***		
2 Lipton® Bedtime Story	✓ Total Fat 1g 2%		
Caffeine-Free Herbal	✓ Saturated Fat 0g	0%	
Pyramid Tea Bags	✓ Trans Fat 0g		
	✓ Cholesterol 0mg	0%	
2 SERVINGS	✓ Sodium 35mg	1%	
TOTAL TIME 8MINS	✓ Potassium	0%	
	✓ Total Carbohydrate 9g 3%		
	✓ Dietary Fiber less than 1g		4%
	✓ Sugars 7g		
	✓ Protein 3g		
	✓ Vitamin A	8%	
	✓ Vitamin C	0%	
	✓ Calcium	2%	
	✓ Iron	4%	

Instructions:

1. Pour boiling water over Lipton® Bedtime Story Caffeine-Free Herbal Pyramid Tea Bags; cover and brew 3 minutes. Remove Tea Bags and squeeze. Stir in sugar until dissolved.

2. Meanwhile, in microwave-safe bowl, microwave milk with cinnamon at HIGH 1 minute or until warm; remove cinnamon. Stir into hot tea and serve immediately.

Caffeine Free Chocolate Devil Food Cake

INGREDIENTS
✓ 2 cups flour
✓ 1 cup sugar
✓ 1 cup Nesquick brand chocolate drink powder (it's 99.9% caffeine-free)
✓ 1/2 cup carob powder
✓ 2 tsp baking soda (divided)
✓ 1/2 tsp salt
✓ 1/2 cup vegetable shortening
✓ 1 1/4 cups milk (divided)
✓ 1 tsp vanilla
✓ 3 eggs
✓ Mayonnaise
2 SERVINGS
TOTAL TIME 65MINS

Instructions:

1. Preheat oven to 350 degrees Fahrenheit.

2. Whisk together flour, sugar, Nesquick, carob powder, 1 tsp baking soda, and salt in a large mixing bowl. Drop in shortening and add 3/4 cup milk and the vanilla. Mix at lowest speed 15 seconds with an electric mixer just to blend.

3. Beat for 2 minutes at medium speed, scraping bowl and beaters as needed (the dough will be the consistency of cookie

dough, thick and sticky, so you will have to do this often to keep the dough from clogging the beaters).

4.   Add the remaining ingredients, minus the mayonnaise, and beat until well blended. Add approximately 3 large tbsp of mayonnaise and beat until it is thoroughly blended. Pour into ungreased cake pan(s) and bake approximately 40-45 minutes or until a knife inserted into the middle comes out clean and the cake is springy to the touch (meaning if you were to press gently on the top of the cake it would regain its shape). Cool in pan for about 5 minutes, then transfer cake to a cooling rack and cool completely.

5.   Fill and frost as desired.

VARIATION : COOKIES

1.   Once the dough becomes the consistency of cookie dough, use a spoon to drop the dough onto a cookie sheet and bake for approximately 15-20 minutes for delicious chocolate cookies instead.

Mint-tea Lemonade

INGREDIENTS	NUTRITION FACTS (Per Serving)		
2 cups boiling water	✓ Calories 80		
2 cups prepared lemonade	✓ Calories from Fat 0		
1 small lemon, sliced			
1/4 cup sugar	**% Daily Value** *		
6 Lipton® Bedtime Story	✓ Total Fat 0g 0%		
Caffeine-Free Herbal	✓ Saturated Fat 0g	0%	
Pyramid Tea Bags	✓ Trans Fat 0g		
	✓ Cholesterol 0mg	0%	
5 SERVINGS	✓ Sodium 10mg	0%	
TOTAL TIME 15MINS	✓ Potassium 0%		
	✓ Total Carbohydrate 23g		8%
	✓ Dietary Fiber less than 1g		4%
	✓ Sugars 20g		
	✓ Protein 0g		
	✓ Vitamin A 0%		
	✓ Vitamin C 35%		
	✓ Calcium 2%		
	✓ Iron 2%		

Instructions:

1. Pour boiling water over Lipton® Bedtime Story Caffeine-Free Herbal Pyramid Tea Bags; cover and brew 5 minutes. Remove Tea Bags and squeeze. Stir in sugar until dissolved; cool.

2. In pitcher, combine all ingredients.

3. Serve over ice.

Iced Raspberry Tea

INGREDIENTS
✓   Gallon water
✓   1 cup sugar
✓   4 decaffeinated black tea bags
✓   2 caffeine free raspberry flavored tea bags
16 SERVINGS
TOTAL TIME 10MINS

Instructions:

1. Bring the water to a boil.

2. Reduce heat to a simmer and mix in sugar. Make sure it's completely dissolved.

3. Begin steeping all tea bags. Steep approximately 8-10 minutes or till desired flavor is achieved.

4. Allow to cool before serving and serve over ice.

5. Store unused tea in fridge.

Egg-free, Sugar-free, Caffeine-free Chocolate Cupcakes

INGREDIENTS

- ✓ 1 cup (150g) self-raising flour
- ✓ ½ cup (100g) firmly packed pitted dates
- ✓ 1/3 cup (100g) rice malt syrup
- ✓ 100g unsalted butter, diced and left out of the fridge for at least 30 minutes before baking
- ✓ 1 teaspoon of natural vanilla extract or vanilla bean paste
- ✓ 1/3 cup of carob powder
- ✓ 1/2 teaspoon bi-carb soda
- ✓ ½ cup milk
- ✓ 2 eggs worth of natural egg replacer
(or just 2 eggs if not allergic)

5 SERVINGS
TOTAL TIME 15MINS

Instructions:

1. Pre-heat a fan-forced oven to 180 degrees and line two cupcake trays with 12 patty cases.

2. Place dates, rice malt syrup, carob powder, vanilla, egg mixture and half the milk into a food processor and blend for at least three minutes, until all the dates are processed and you have a smooth chocolate mixture as shown below. The longer the better when it comes to the time they are blending in the food processor.

3. While the date mixture is combining in the food processor, cream the butter in a large bowl with an electric beater for five minutes. Stop halfway to scrape any butter back into the centre of the bowl that might have escaped up the sides.

4. In a separate, smaller bowl sift the flour and bi-carb soda together.

5. Slowly add sifted flour and chocolate mixture to the creamed butter in alternate batches. Beating each time until just combined.

6. Add remaining milk to the mixture and beat until just combined.

7. Spoon mixture into patty cases and fill to around half to three-quarters full depending on how big you want the cupcakes.

8. Place in oven for 15-20 minutes or until a skewer inserted into the centre of the cupcake comes out clean. Check at 15 minutes if they are cooked as you don't want to over bake.

9. Allow to cool for a few minutes in the tray before transferring to a wire rack to cool completely.

10. Pipe or spread on my sugar-free chocolate cream cheese frosting or my sugar-free raspberry cream cheese frosting.

Blueberry-Coconut Baked Steel Cut Oatmeal

INGREDIENTS

- ✓ 1 1/2 cups (260 grams) Steel Cut Irish Oats
- ✓ 1/2 teaspoon ground Ginger
- ✓ 1/2 teaspoon fine Sea Salt
- ✓ 1 teaspoon Baking Powder
- ✓ 4 cups (950 ml, 32 ounces) unsweetened Vanilla Almond Milk
- ✓ 2 cups (480 ml, 16 ounces) light unsweetened Coconut Milk
- ✓ 1 1/2 (240 grams) cups fresh Blueberries
(frozen OK too, do not thaw first)
- ✓ 1/4 cup (47 grams) unsweetened dried Blueberries
- ✓ 1/4 cup (22 grams) unsweetened Coconut Flake
- ✓ Vanilla Stevia Drops or your favorite natural sweetener to taste

- ✓ Blueberry Sauce
- ✓ 2 cups (360 grams) fresh or frozen Blueberries

- ✓ Optional Toppings
- ✓ Toasted Nuts
- ✓ Coconut Flake
- ✓ Whipped Cream (vegan or not)
- ✓ extra dried and fresh Blueberries
- ✓ Coconut Milk

8 SERVINGS
TOTAL TIME 65MINS

Instructions:

OATMEAL

1. Pre heat oven to 350 degrees F with the rack in the center. Lightly coat a 13X9X2" inch baking dish with cooking spray. Combine all ingredients in a large bowl adding blueberries and coconut last. Sweeten to taste (I used 2 droppers full of vanilla stevia drops.) Bake for about one hour. The oatmeal will appear not done when you take it out of the oven. Remove from the oven and let it cool to room temperature. Then put it in your refrigerator overnight for best results. It will thicken nicely in there.

BLUEBERRY SAUCE

1. Heat the blueberries with a splash of water over medium high heat. When you hear them sizzle reduce heat to medium and cook for about 5 minutes until saucy. Mash the blueberries against the side of the pan with a spatula.

2. Serve oatmeal with some almond or coconut milk and blueberry sauce.

3. Notes

4.   Cook this oatmeal the night before you plan on serving it so it has time to thicken in the refrigerator. Re-heat portions before serving.

Chicken, Veggie, Avocado and Rice Bowls

INGREDIENTS

Chicken
- ✓ 1 pound boneless skinless chicken breast or tenders, cubed if using skewers, leave whole if not
- ✓ 1/4 cup olive oil
- ✓ 4 cloves garlic, minced or grated
- ✓ 1/2 teaspoon onion powder
- ✓ 1/2 teaspoon pepper
- ✓ 1/4 teaspoon cayenne
- ✓ 1/2 teaspoon smoked paprika
- ✓ 1/4 cup fresh parsley, chopped (may sub 1 tablespoon dried)
- ✓ 1/4 cup fresh basil, chopped (may sub 1 tablespoon dried)

The Rice + Veggies + Avocado
- ✓ 1 1/2 cups jasmine or basmati rice
- ✓ 3 cups water
- ✓ 2 red pepper, cut into fourths
- ✓ 1 zucchini, sliced into 1/4 inch rounds
- ✓ 1 tablespoon olive oil
- ✓ salt + pepper
- ✓ 2 avocados, mashed very well
- ✓ juice of 1 lemon
- ✓ 1/2 cup fresh parsley, chopped
- ✓ 1 clove garlic, minced or grated
- ✓ salt + pepper, to taste
- ✓ 1 pint grape tomatoes, halved
- ✓ 1/4 cup walnuts, toasted
- ✓ 1/2 cup blue cheese, crumbled (optional)

4 SERVINGS
TOTAL TIME 50MINS

Instructions:

1. At least 30 minutes before grilling, soak your skewers (if they are bamboo) in water for 30 minutes to prevent them from charring. In a large bowl combine the olive oil, garlic, onion powder, pepper, cayenne, smoked paprika, parsley and basil.

2. Add the chicken and toss well. Cover and place in the fridge while you prepare the rest of the meal. Make the rice.

3. Add the water to a medium size pot.

4. Bring to a low boil and then add the rice. Stir to combine and then place the lid on the pot and turn the heat down to the lowest setting possible.

5. Allow the rice to cook ten minutes on low and then turn the heat off completely and let the rice sit on the stove, covered for another 20 minutes (don't take any peeks inside!).

6. After 20 minutes remove the lid and fluff the rice with a fork. Note that rice can cook differently for everyone, this is just what works for me. Pre heat the grill to medium high heat. Add the red pepper and zucchini to a gallon size Ziploc bag.

7. Add 1 tablespoon of olive oil and a pinch of salt and pepper. Seal the bag and shake well so the veggies are coated with olive oil. Remove the chicken from the fridge and if using skewers, skewer the chicken (or if you do not have skewers you can leave the chicken whole and cut after grilling).

8.   Grill the chicken for 3-4 minutes per side, gently flipping 2-3 times until chicken is cooked through and has light char marks. While the chicken is grilling grill the zucchini for about 4 minutes on each side, or until tender and the red peppers for about 5 minutes flipping once or twice during cooking. You may also use a grill pan to do this or even just cook everything on the stove. Remove everything from the grill and let cool 5 minutes. Once cool slice the red peppers into strips and if you have whole chicken breast cut those into cubes. Add the mashed avocados to a bowl.

9.   Stir in the lemon juice, parsley, garlic and salt and pepper to taste. Mix well. To assemble the bowls, divide the rice among 4 bowls or plates. Top each bowl of rice with equal amounts of chicken, grilled peppers and zucchini. Add a large dollop of the avocados and then add the fresh tomatoes and walnuts. Sprinkle with blue cheese if desired. Serve warm.

Detox Rainbow Salad

INGREDIENTS	NUTRITION FACTS (Per Serving)		
2 C. Rainbow Slaw, Dry	✓	Calories	245.8
2 C. Romaine, Chopped	✓	Fat	17.2g
1/2 Medium Red Bell Pepper, Diced	✓	Carb	24.7g
1 Avocado	✓	Fiber	13.5g
2 Tsp. Sesame Seeds	✓	Protein	7.9g
Salt & Pepper to Taste	✓	Sugar	7.7g
	✓	Sodium	62.5mg
2 SERVINGS TOTAL TIME 50MINS			

Instructions:

1. Combine the slaw, romaine and red bell together in a large bowl.

Pumpkin-Lentil Soup With A Maca Boost

INGREDIENTS
✓   2 cups lentils (preferably soaked in water overnight)
✓   6 cups water
✓   1 cup full fat coconut milk
✓   1 small sugar pumpkin, peeled
✓   1 tsp. curry powder
✓   1/2 tsp. garlic powder
✓   1/4 tsp. ginger powder
✓   2 Tbsp. chopped basil
✓   2 Tbsp. chopped sage
✓   2 Tbsp. maca powder
✓   1 tsp. mesquite powder (optional)
✓   1 head kale, chopped
✓   1/2 tsp (or more) sea salt
✓   pepper, to taste
TOTAL TIME 30MINS

Instructions:

1. Add every ingredient except kale to the pot. Bring to a boil, reduce to simmer, and cover. Keep this on the stove for at least a couple hours. The longer the better; the flavors infuse more and more with each minute that goes by.

2. When you're getting ready to serve, add the kale. Let the soup heat the kale to the point at which it turns just green, approximately three minutes.

3. Top your soup with fresh basil and fresh sprouts for some raw goodness!

4. As always, sit in gratitude and love before eating your meal. Feel the radiance of the light and spirit within you, on your plate, in your life, and then you may begin.

5. Enjoy the heck out of it!

Fall Mexican Rice Bowls

INGREDIENTS

For the Rice:

- ✓ 1 1/4 cup uncooked basmati rice
- ✓ 2 cups water
- ✓ 1/2 cup salsa
- ✓ 1/2 of a purple onion, diced
- ✓ 8 ounces peeled and diced sweet potato
- ✓ 1/2 teaspoon cumin
- ✓ 3/4 teaspoon chili powder
- ✓ 3.5 ounces chopped kale
- ✓ 1 can Bush's Kidney Beans, drained
- ✓ 1 can Bush's Black Beans, drained
- ✓ salt and pepper, to taste

For the Chicken:

- ✓ 1 lb. boneless, skinless chicken breasts, cubed
- ✓ salt and pepper, to taste
- ✓ 1/2 teaspoon cumin
- ✓ 1/2 teaspoon chili powder

[Optional - or use leftover meat from a previous night's dinner or rotisserie chicken]

- ✓ Topping Ideas:
- ✓ Lime Wedges
- ✓ Avocado Slices
- ✓ Salsa
- ✓ Shredded Pepper Jack Cheese

6 SERVINGS

TOTAL TIME 30MINS

Instructions:

1. In a saucepan, add the water, salsa, and rice. Bring the mixture to a boil, cover with a lid, and turn the heat all the way to low. Allow to cook for 15 minutes.

2. Meanwhile, in a large cast iron skillet or stainless steel pan, heat 2 teaspoons of olive oil. Add the diced onion and sauté for 5-7 minutes, or until tender.

3. Then add the sweet potato, cumin, and chili powder and sauté until the sweet potatoes are tender. Add the chopped kale and cook just until wilted. Stir in the beans. Turn heat to low and set aside while you prepare the chicken.

4. Heat 2 teaspoons of olive oil in a cast iron skillet or stainless steel pan. Add the chicken and seasonings and cook until the chicken is done. Set aside.

5. In a large bowl (or your skillet if it is large enough), combine the cooked rice with the vegetables.

6. To serve, scoop the rice and vegetable mixture into bowls, top with cubed chicken. Although not necessary, serve with any toppings that you prefer.

NOTES:

- This recipe is very forgiving. You can easily swap out vegetables according to season or personal preference. Other great vegetable additions or substitutions include red bell pepper, sliced mushrooms, diced butternut squash, spinach, or tomatoes.

- If you like extra heat, try including fire roasted green chilies or minced chipotle peppers in adobo sauce in the rice.

- Vegetarian option may omit the chicken.

- A variety of rice can be used as well. If your family prefers brown rice, that is a suitable substitute. Quinoa is another great grain substitution.

Green Goddess Enchiladas

INGREDIENTS

✓   1 cup dried chickpeas, soaked overnight
and boiled in salted water until tender

✓   1 small onion, diced

✓   1 (10 oz) can Ro-tel diced tomatoes and chilies

✓   1 cup frozen corn

✓   1/2 tsp dried oregano

✓   kosher salt and black pepper

✓   1 cup grated reduced fat cheddar cheese (I used Cabot)

✓   10-12 corn tortillas

✓   1 3/4 cup low sodium vegetable broth

✓   1 cup nonfat Greek yogurt

✓   1 bunch kale, stemmed

✓   1 (4 oz) can green chilies

✓   2 scallions, chopped

6 SERVINGS

Instructions:

1.   In a large nonstick skillet, spray with cooking spray and, over medium-low heat, sauté chickpeas, onion, Ro-tel, corn, oregano, 1 teaspoon salt and 1/8 teaspoon black pepper. Sauté 5-6 minutes over medium-low heat or until all liquid from tomatoes has evaporated, stirring often. Remove from heat.

2.   In a blender or food processor, puree the vegetable broth, Greek yogurt, kale, chilies, and scallions.

3. Preheat oven to 400 degrees F. Grease a 9×13 casserole or baking dish. Lightly cover bottom of the dish with 1/2-3/4 cup of the sauce.

4. Heat corn tortillas by wrapping the stack of them in aluminum foil and placing them in the preheating oven for 5-7 minutes or by microwaving them covered with a wet paper towel for 30 seconds.

5. Stir 1/2 cup of cheese into the chickpea mixture. Add heaping 1/2 cups of filling to one end of each tortilla and roll up or fold in half placing each one seam side down in the prepared casserole dish.

6. Pour kale sauce evenly over top of enchiladas. It will be very liquid, but don't worry, it will thicken as it cooks. Sprinkle remaining 1/2 cup of cheese over the enchiladas. Bake for about 25 minutes until bubbly all over. Allow to sit for five minutes before serving.

No Grain, No Problem Recipes

Eliminating grain in your diet will do a lot. It's going to activate our thyroid hormone as well as reset insulin and leptin.

Simple Cabbage Soup

INGREDIENTS
Olive oil and butter
✓   1 large onion, coarsely chopped
✓   3-5 stalks celery, sliced
✓   3 carrots, sliced
✓   4 cloves garlic, chopped
✓   1-2 cans great northern beans
✓   ½ head cabbage, thinly sliced
✓   6 cups chicken stock
✓   1-2 cups pumpkin
✓   1 tsp salt
✓   ½ tsp pepper
✓   1+ tsp cumin
6-8 SERVINGS
TOTAL TIME 40MINS

Instructions:

1. Melt 1Tbs butter and 2Tbs olive oil.

2. Add the onion, celery, carrots, garlic, and beans in order as you chop them.

3. By the time you add the beans, the onions should be soft.

4. Add salt, pepper, cumin and stir.

5. Add cabbage and cover 5 minutes or so to wilt.

6. Add broth, pumpkin (frozen is fine) and optional tomato sauce.

7. Bring to a boil and reduce to high simmer.

8. Cover and cook 15-30 minutes until carrots and cabbage are tender.

No Gluten Wanton Soup

INGREDIENTS	NUTRITION FACTS (Per Serving)	
13/4 cups gluten free all purpose flour (I used Better Batter, plus more for sprinkling)	✓ Calories 5	
	✓ Calories from Fat 0	
3/4 tsp xanthan gum (omit if your blend already contains it)	**% Daily Value ***	
	✓ Total Fat 0g 0%	
35 grams tapioca starch (Expanded modified)	✓ Saturated Fat 0g	0%
	✓ Trans Fat	
3 eggs (180g, out of shell at room temperature, beaten)	✓ Cholesterol 10mg	3%
	✓ Sodium 0mg 0%	
6 tbsps warm water (about 85°F)	✓ Potassium 0mg	0%
	✓ Total Carbohydrate	
	less than 1g 0%	
6 SERVINGS	✓ Dietary Fiber	0%
TOTAL TIME 35MINS	✓ Sugars 0g	
	✓ Protein 0g	
	✓ Vitamin A 0%	
	✓ Vitamin C 0%	
	✓ Calcium 0%	
	✓ Iron 0%	

Instructions:

1. In the bowl of a stand mixer fitted with the paddle attachment (or a large bowl with a wooden spoon), place the flour, xanthan gum and Expanded, and whisk to combine well with a separate handheld whisk.

2. Create a well in the center of the dry ingredients, and add the eggs and 4 tablespoons warm water, and mix to combine on medium speed for about 1 minute (or with the wooden spoon for at least 2 minutes). The dough should come together. If there are any crumbly bits, add the remaining warm water by the teaspoon until the dough holds together well when squeezed with your hands.

3. Turn the mixer speed up to medium-high, and beat until smooth, 3 to 4 minutes (or by hand with a wooden spoon for at least twice as long). The dough should be smooth and pliable. If it feels stiff, add a few more drops of water and mix in until pliable. It should be, at most, slightly sticky but mostly just smooth.

4. Transfer the dough to a piece of plastic wrap, wrap it tightly and allow it to sit at room temperature for about 10 minutes. The dough will absorb more water and any remaining stickiness should dissipate. Unwrap the dough, divide it in half and return half of it to the plastic wrap and wrap tightly

to prevent it from drying out. Place the remaining half of the dough on a lightly floured surface, sprinkle lightly with more flour and roll into a rectangle about 1/4-inch thick.

5. Flip and shift the dough often to prevent it from sticking, sprinkling very lightly with more flour as necessary to allow movement. With a pizza wheel, pastry cutter or sharp knife, trim the edges of the rectangle to create even edges. Remove and gather the trimmings, and set them aside.

6. Using even and sustained, but not aggressive, pressure, roll out the rectangle until it is approximately 1/8 inch thick. Slice into 3-inch squares. Alternatively, slice the 1/4-inch thick rectangle into 1 1/2-inch squares, and roll each square evenly in all directions until it doubles in surface area and is 1/8-inch thick. I often find this the quicker, easier way to get squares that are the proper thickness.

7. Use wonton wrappers in gluten free eggrolls, gluten free crab rangoon, or wonton dumplings for soup. Stack any leftover wrappers, wrap first in waxed paper and then place in a freezer-safe container, seal tightly and freeze until ready to use. Defrost by placing overnight in the refrigerator before using. Add salt, pepper, cumin and stir.

8. Add cabbage and cover 5 minutes or so to wilt.

9. Add broth, pumpkin (frozen is fine) and optional tomato sauce.

10. Bring to a boil and reduce to high simmer.

11. Cover and cook 15-30 minutes until carrots and cabbage are tender.

Grain Free Pancakes

INGREDIENTS	NUTRITION FACTS (Per Serving)		
125 grams gluten-free flour	✓ Calories 280		
1 egg	✓ Calories from Fat 110		
250 ml low-fat milk (or your preference of milk)	**% Daily Value ***		
Butter (for frying)	✓ Total Fat 12g	18%	
	✓ Saturated Fat 7g	35%	
3 SERVINGS	✓ Trans Fat		
TOTAL TIME 25MINS	✓ Cholesterol 95mg	32%	
	✓ Sodium 120mg	5%	
	✓ Potassium 270mg	8%	
	✓ Total Carbohydrate 36g		12%
	✓ Dietary Fiber 2g	8%	
	✓ Sugars 5g		
	✓ Protein 8g		
	✓ Vitamin A	10%	
	✓ Vitamin C	0%	
	✓ Calcium	10%	
	✓ Iron	6%	

Instructions:

1. Start by putting the flour into a small mixing bowl and making a small 'well' in the centre. Crack the egg in the middle and pour in the contents along with a quarter of the milk.

2. Use an electric or hand whisk to thoroughly combine the mixture. When it turns into a paste, mix in another quarter of the milk.

3. Once it's smooth and lump free, mix in what's left of the milk and leave to stand for 20 minutes.

4. Heat a knob of butter in a small non-stick frying pan. Then, when the butter starts to foam, pour a small amount of mixture into the pan and swirl around until it covers the base.

5. Cook your pancake for a few minutes until golden brown then flip over and cook the other side until it's the same color.

6. Carry on until you've used all the mixture. You may need to add a little more butter between frying. Your delicious gluten free pancakes are now ready to serve and how you serve them depends on how you like them.

7. Traditionalists would go for a squeeze of lemon juice and a sprinkling of sugar, but a little syrup also goes down very nicely. You could even turn them into savory pancakes with the filling of your choice.

Tropical Mango Spinach Smoothie

INGREDIENTS	NUTRITION FACTS (Per Serving)	
1 mango (chopped)	✓ Calories 320	
1 bananas (chopped)	✓ Calories from Fat 0	
1 cup spinach (chopped, loosely packed)	**% Daily Value ***	
3/4 cup coconut water	✓ Total Fat	0%
2 tsps honey	✓ Saturated Fat	0%
	✓ Trans Fat	
	✓ Cholesterol	0%
1 SERVING	✓ Sodium 220mg	9%
TOTAL TIME 15MINS	✓ Potassium 1370mg	39%
	✓ Total Carbohydrate	
	82g 27%	
	✓ Dietary Fiber 10g	40%
	✓ Sugars 62g	
	✓ Protein 6g	
	✓ Vitamin A 90%	
	✓ Vitamin C 140%	
	✓ Calcium 10%	
	✓ Iron 6%	

Instructions:

1. Add mango, banana, coconut water and honey in a blender and give a good spin till everything is blended well and you get a thick smooth consistency.

2. Pour half of the smoothie in glass.

3. Now add spinach to the rest of the smoothie in the blender and blitz till smoothie is bright green in color. Add some coconut water if required.

4. Fill rest of the glass with it and slurp.

Cheesy Broccoli Casserole

INGREDIENTS	NUTRITION FACTS (Per Serving)		
2 tbsps butter (dairy or non dairy, We like Earth Balance)	✓ Calories 270		
2 tbsps gluten free all purpose flour (we use Better Batter)	✓ Calories from Fat 190		
2 cups milk (dairy or non dairy)	**% Daily Value ***		
4 oz. cream cheese (diced, dairy or non dairy, We like tofutti)	✓ Total Fat 21g	32%	
1/3 cup shredded cheese (your choice)	✓ Saturated Fat 12g	60%	
12 oz. frozen hash browns	✓ Trans Fat		
2 cups broccoli (steamed)	✓ Cholesterol 65mg	22%	
	✓ Sodium 280mg	12%	
4 SERVINGs	✓ Potassium 420mg	12%	
TOTAL TIME 55MINS	✓ Total Carbohydrate 11g		4%
	✓ Dietary Fiber 1g	4%	
	✓ Sugars 8g		
	✓ Protein 10g		
	✓ Vitamin A 20%		
	✓ Vitamin C 70%		
	✓ Calcium 30%		
	✓ Iron 4%		

Instructions:

1. Preheat oven to 350 degrees F.

2. In a large pan, melt butter and stir in flour.

3. Next add milk and cheese. Stir until melted.

4. Add potatoes and heat thoroughly.

5. Add steamed broccoli, stir.

6. Pour into prepared (lightly oiled) casserole dish.

7. Bake for 20 to 35 minutes; or until browned.

8. Enjoy.

Gluten Free BBQ Casserole Bites

INGREDIENTS	NUTRITION FACTS (Per Serving)		
1 cup chicken (chopped)	✓ Calories 340		
1 cup broccoli (chopped)	✓ Calories from Fat 110		
1 cup shredded cheese			
1 cup wild rice (cooked)	**% Daily Value ***		
1 eggs	✓ Total Fat 13g	20%	
	✓ Saturated Fat 7g	35%	
	✓ Trans Fat		
4 SERVINGS	✓ Cholesterol 120mg	40%	
TOTAL TIME 30MINS	✓ Sodium 250mg	10%	
	✓ Potassium 420mg	12%	
	✓ Total Carbohydrate 32g		11%
	✓ Dietary Fiber 3g	12%	
	✓ Sugars 2g		
	✓ Protein 27g		
	✓ Vitamin A 10%		
	✓ Vitamin C 35%		
	✓ Calcium 25%		
	✓ Iron 10%		

Instructions:

1. Preheat oven to 350.

2. Combine all the ingredients in a bowl and then scoop into a greased muffin tin.

3. Bake for 20 minutes.

Mexican Baked Brown Rice

INGREDIENTS	NUTRITION FACTS (Per Serving)	
2 cooked chicken breasts (shredded)	✓ Calories 370	
1 cup brown rice	✓ Calories from Fat 100	
1 cup refried beans		
3/4 cup enchilada sauce	**% Daily Value ***	
1 cup shredded cheese	✓ Total Fat 11g	17%
1/2 green pepper (diced)	✓ Saturated Fat 6g	30%
2 tsps chili flakes (optional)	✓ Trans Fat	
	✓ Cholesterol 30mg	10%
4 SERVINGS	✓ Sodium 840mg	35%
TOTAL TIME 30MINS	✓ Potassium 380mg	11%
	✓ Total Carbohydrate	
	51g 17%	
	✓ Dietary Fiber 6g	24%
	✓ Sugars 4g	
	✓ Protein 15g	
	✓ Vitamin A 20%	
	✓ Vitamin C 30%	
	✓ Calcium 25%	
	✓ Iron 15%	

Instructions:

1. Cook brown rice. You can use a rice cooker or you can manually do it using a pot.

2. Heat oven to 350and grease a 9x9 baking dish.

3. In a mixing bowl, stir together the shredded chicken and enchilada sauce. Mix in the rice and beans and stir until it's all combined.

4. Transfer the mixture to the prepared 9x9 dish and top with the green peppers, then the shredded cheese and chili flakes.

5. Bake for 25-30 minutes, then broil for 2-3 to get a bit of crispiness to the layer of cheese.

Corn Tortillas

INGREDIENTS	NUTRITION FACTS (Per Serving)	
2 cups masa harina	✓ Calories 210	
11/4 cups warm water	✓ Calories from Fat 20	
1 tsp arrowroot powder		
(tapioca starch – gluten-free)	**% Daily Value ***	
	✓ Total Fat 2.5g	4%
	✓ Saturated Fat 0.5g	3%
4 SERVINGS	✓ Trans Fat	
TOTAL TIME 30MINS	✓ Cholesterol 0%	
	✓ Sodium 5mg 0%	
	✓ Potassium 170mg	5%
	✓ Total Carbohydrate 44g	15%
	✓ Dietary Fiber 6g	24%
	✓ Sugars less than 1g	
	✓ Protein 5g	
	✓ Vitamin A 0%	
	✓ Vitamin C 0%	
	✓ Calcium 8%	
	✓ Iron 20%	

Instructions:

1. Use a wooden bowl to combine the masa harina and water. Mix well until the water is absorbed evenly and the dough forms a ball.

2. We are looking for a soft dough consistency; it should not stick to your hands. If it does, add a little more masa harina. If it looks dry, breakable or crumbly, add more water.

3. Preheat a griddle or heavy skillet on medium flame. This has to be ready when you start pressing the tortillas.

4. Using a tortilla press or a heavy dish, place a ball of the dough between the two plastic pieces and press to form a flat 10-12 cm round tortilla.

5. Open the tortilla press or remove the heavy dish (if using to press the tortillas), peel the top plastic off.

6. Place the tortilla on the griddle and cook for 45 seconds. The edge will begin to dry out. Turn over and continue to cook for 1 minute until brown patches form. The cooking time is about 2 minutes total. Cook until the tortilla begins to puff. Tap lightly with your fingertips to allow even puffing.

7. Fill with your favorite ingredients and serve warm.

Vanilla Latte Martini

INGREDIENTS	NUTRITION FACTS (Per Serving)	
3 oz. vanilla vodka	✓ Calories 110	
2 oz. coffee liqueur (homemade)	✓ Calories from Fat 15	
1 tbsp cream		
	% Daily Value *	
	✓ Total Fat 1.5g	2%
2 SERVINGS	✓ Saturated Fat 1g	5%
TOTAL TIME 10MINS	✓ Trans Fat	
	✓ Cholesterol less than 5 mg	2%
	✓ Sodium 5mg 0%	
	✓ Potassium 20mg	1%
	✓ Total Carbohydrate 14g	5%
	✓ Dietary Fiber	0%
	✓ Sugars 13g	
	✓ Protein 0g	
	✓ Vitamin A	2%
	✓ Vitamin C	0%
	✓ Calcium	2%
	✓ Iron	0%

Instructions:

1. Fill a cocktail shaker with ice. Add coffee liqueur, vanilla vodka and cream. Shake well and divide between two chilled martini glasses.

NOTES: Serves 2. Each serving has 3.6 g of carbs.

Chocolate Avocado Truffle

INGREDIENTS	NUTRITION FACTS (Per Serving)	
1 avocado (large ripe)	✓ Calories 60	
1/4 cup Dutch-processed cocoa powder (+ extra for dusting)	✓ Calories from Fat 35	
1/4 cup powdered sugar	**% Daily Value ***	
1/4 cup pumpkin seeds	✓ Total Fat 4g	6%
(chopped, for rolling, optional)	✓ Saturated Fat 0.5g	3%
	✓ Trans Fat	
	✓ Cholesterol 0%	
12 SERVINGS	✓ Sodium 0mg	0%
TOTAL TIME 25MINS	✓ Potassium 150mg	4%
	✓ Total Carbohydrate 6g	2%
	✓ Dietary Fiber 2g	8%
	✓ Sugars 3g	
	✓ Protein 1g	
	✓ Vitamin A	0%
	✓ Vitamin C	4%
	✓ Calcium	2%
	✓ Iron	4%

Instructions:

1. If you using pumpkin seeds, chop in a food processor until a crushed "nut" consistency. Set aside. Clean processor.

2.   Puree avocado until smooth. Add in sugar and cocoa powder and mix until blended.

3.   Using a cookie scoop, gently drop and roll balls into coating of choice.

4.   Serve and enjoy right away.

Freedom from Dairy Recipes

It doesn't matter if you're not lactose intolerant. Erasing dairy from your diet will reset your growth hormone which, as a result, also improves insulin.

Blueberry Baked Oatmeal

INGREDIENTS	NUTRITION FACTS (Per Serving)	
2 cups gluten-free rolled oats	✓ Calories 270	
shredded coconut (or 1 cup	✓ Calories from Fat 140	
unsweetened flaked, optional)		
11/2 tsps baking powder	**% Daily Value ***	
1/4 tsp ground cinnamon	✓ Total Fat 15g	23%
3/4 tsp sea salt	✓ Saturated Fat 12g	60%
3 eggs (lightly beaten)	✓ Trans Fat	
2 cups coconut milk	✓ Cholesterol 70mg	23%
(Pacific Foods)	✓ Sodium 230mg	10%
1 tsp vanilla extract	✓ Potassium 270mg	8%
1 cup pure maple syrup	✓ Total Carbohydrate 33g	11%
2 cups frozen blueberries	✓ Dietary Fiber 2g	8%
	✓ Sugars 27g	
9 SERVINGS	✓ Protein 4g	
TOTAL TIME 70MINS	✓ Vitamin A 2%	
	✓ Vitamin C 8%	
	✓ Calcium 10%	
	✓ Iron 10%	

Instructions:

1. Preheat the oven to 350 degrees F. Lightly oil a 8" x 8" baking dish.

2. Stir together the rolled oats, coconut, baking powder, cinnamon and sea salt in a mixing bowl.

3. Whisk together the eggs, coconut milk, vanilla extract, and maple syrup in a separate mixing bowl. Add the oat mixture

to the bowl with the wet mixture and stir well to combine. Stir in the frozen blueberries and pour the mixture into the prepared baking dish.

4. Place on the center rack of the oven and bake for 55 to 65 minutes, or until oatmeal has set up and is cooked through.

5. Remove from the oven and allow baked oatmeal to cool 20 to 30 minutes before serving (Note: if you don't allow the oatmeal to sit after it comes out of the oven, it will fall apart).

Green Tea Breakfast Smoothie

INGREDIENTS	NUTRITION FACTS (Per Serving)		
1 container Silk Vanilla Dairy-Free Yogurt Alternative	✓ Calories 360		
1 cup green tea, brewed and chilled	✓ Calories from Fat 120		
1/4 c + 1 Tbsp honey	**% Daily Value ***		
almond protein granola	✓ Total Fat 13g	20%	
1/2 cup frozen blueberries	✓ Saturated Fat 1g	5%	
	✓ Trans Fat 0g		
	✓ Cholesterol 0mg	0%	
	✓ Sodium 135mg	6%	
1 SERVING	✓ Potassium 0%		
TOTAL TIME 5MINS	✓ Total Carbohydrate 46g		15%
	✓ Dietary Fiber 8g	32%	
	✓ Sugars		
	✓ Protein 19g		
	✓ Vitamin A 0%		
	✓ Vitamin C 2%		
	✓ Calcium 25000%		
	✓ Iron 20000%		

Instructions:

1. Blend all ingredients until creamy and prepare to seize the day!

Creamy Dairy Free Tomato Soup

INGREDIENTS	NUTRITION FACTS (Per Serving)		
1 tbsp canola oil (or oil of choice)	✓	Calories 80	
1/2 cup diced onions	✓	Calories from Fat 20	
1 stick celery (chopped)			
1 carrots (medium, chopped)	**% Daily Value ***		
1 clove garlic (chopped)	✓	Total Fat 2.5g	4%
796 ml diced tomatoes	✓	Saturated Fat 0g	0%
(no salt added)	✓	Trans Fat	
1 potatoes (medium,	✓	Cholesterol	0%
peeled and diced)	✓	Sodium 790mg	33%
11/2 cups gluten-free	✓	Potassium 520mg	15%
vegetable stock (chicken	✓	Total Carbohydrate 14g	5%
stock can be substituted)	✓	Dietary Fiber 3g	12%
2 tsps salt (less if your diced	✓	Sugars 6g	
tomatoes contain salt)	✓	Protein 2g	
1 tsp parsley (or 1 tablespoon fresh)	✓	Vitamin A	60%
1 tsp granulated sugar	✓	Vitamin C	45%
1/2 tsp ground black pepper	✓	Calcium 4%	
	Iron	2%	
6 SERVINGS			
TOTAL TIME 45MINS			

Instructions:

1. In a large pot over medium heat, sauté the onion, celery, carrot, and garlic in the oil until tender, about 10 minutes.

2. Add the remaining ingredients and bring to a boil. Reduce heat and simmer until vegetables are tender, about 20 minutes.

3.   Use an immersion blender to puree the mixture until smooth, or ladle a small amount into a blender and blend until smooth. If you are using a blender or food processor, only work with small amounts of soup at a time. Too much hot liquid in your blender may cause the top to blow off while blending. That's a horrible mess to clean up.

4.   Serve with gluten-free croutons, or gluten-free grilled cheese sticks. Enjoy!

Altamura Pea Soup

INGREDIENTS	NUTRITION FACTS (Per Serving)	
Olive oil	✓ Calories	384
2 medium onions, peeled	✓ Carbs	58.6g
and finely chopped	✓ Sugar	10.7g
4 large handfuls freshly	✓ Fat	8.4g
podded peas	✓ Saturates	1.6g
1.1 liters organic chicken stock	✓ Protein	17.1g
255 g dried spaghetti, broken		
into about 2.5cm lengths		
Sea salt		
Freshly ground black pepper		
1 sprig of fresh mint, optional		
1 sprig of fresh basil, optional		
1 sprig of fresh rosemary, optional		
Extra virgin olive oil		
1 small handful of fresh flat-		
leaf parsley, chopped		
4 SERVINGS		
TOTAL TIME 40MINS		

Instructions:

1. Pour a good lug of olive oil into a pan, add the onions and fry slowly for 10 minutes.

2. Stir in the peas and chicken stock, bring to the boil and simmer for another 10 minutes or so.

3. Bring some salted water to the boil and cook your spaghetti for half the time it says on the packet, then drain and add it to the pea soup to finish cooking.

4. It's nice to tie up the sprigs of herbs and pop them into the soup to give it a lovely fragrance, removing them before serving.

5. When the pasta is cooked, have a taste of the soup and season carefully with salt and pepper.

6. Divide the soup between the bowls, drizzle over a little extra virgin olive oil and sprinkle with the parsley.

NOTE: If using fresh peas, boil up the stock with the shells of the peas. You can do this while you're frying the onions. Then you can strain the stock onto your onions and peas when they're ready and fill the pan up again with water to boil your spaghetti while the soup simmers.

Salmon Fishcakes

INGREDIENTS	NUTRITION FACTS (Per Serving)	
Sea salt and freshly ground black pepper	✓ Calories	383
50 g fresh or frozen peas	✓ Carbs	31.9g
600 g potatoes	✓ Sugar	1.5g
½ a bunch of fresh chives	✓ Fat	16.5g
2 x 180g tins of quality salmon	✓ Saturates	2.8g
1 lemon	✓ Protein	25g
1 tablespoon plain flour, plus extra for dusting		
1 large free-range egg		
Olive oil		
4 SERVINGS TOTAL TIME 90MINS		

Instructions:

1. Half-fill a large saucepan with cold water and add a tiny pinch of salt.

2. Place on a high heat and bring to the boil. Meanwhile…

3. If using fresh peas, pod them into a bowl, then leave to one side.

4. Use a Y-shaped peeler to peel the potatoes, then chop into 1cm chunks on a chopping board.

5. Once the water is boiling, carefully add the potatoes, bring back to the boil, then turn the heat down to medium and simmer gently for around 10 minutes, or until cooked through, adding the peas for the last 2 minutes. Meanwhile...

6. Finely chop the chives and add them to a mixing bowl.

7. Drain the salmon in a sieve over the sink .

8. Add the salmon to the bowl, using a fork to flake it into small chunks.

9. Once cooked, drain the potatoes and peas in a colander over the sink then leave them to cool completely. Meanwhile...

10. Use a micro plane to finely grate the lemon zest, then add it to the bowl along with the flour.

11. Crack in the egg and season with a tiny pinch of pepper.

12. Once cool, tip the potatoes and peas back into the pan and use a potato masher to mash them really well.

13. Add the mash to the bowl, then mix together until really well combined.

14. Sprinkle a little flour over a clean work surface and onto a large plate.

15. Divide the mixture into 8 and use your hands to pat and shape each ball into a fishcake, roughly 2cm thick.

16. Place them onto the floured plate, dusting your hands and the top of each fish cake lightly with flour as you go.

17. Place a large frying pan on a medium heat and add 1 tablespoon of olive oil.

18. Carefully place the fishcakes into the pan and cook for 3 to 4 minutes on each side, or until crisp and golden, turning carefully with a fish slice.

19. Cut the zested lemon into wedges.

20. Serve the fishcakes with some seasonal green veg or a fresh green salad and lemon wedges for squeezing over.

Beef & Broccoli Stir-fry

INGREDIENTS	NUTRITION FACTS (Per Serving)		
200 g purple sprouting broccoli	✓	Calories	427
Sea salt	✓	Carbs	26.5g
Freshly ground black pepper	✓	Sugar	2.3g
2 x 300 g quality sirloin steaks	✓	Fat	17.1g
2 teaspoons coriander seeds	✓	Saturates	5.4g
Olive oil	✓	Protein	39.4g
1 red onion, peeled and finely sliced			
2 cloves garlic peeled and finely sliced			
1 thumb-sized piece fresh ginger, peeled and finely chopped			
3 tablespoons soy sauce			
1 teaspoon sesame oil			
Egg noodles, to serve			
Red chili, finely sliced, to serve			
1 wedge of lime, to serve			
4 SERVINGS TOTAL TIME 25MINS			

Instructions:

1.   Place the broccoli spears into a heatproof bowl and cover them with boiling water. Add a good pinch of salt and leave for 10 minutes. Drain and put to one side.

2.   Slice the steaks into finger-sized strips and season with salt and pepper. Pound the coriander seeds in a pestle and mortar, then sprinkle over the meat so they stick to it and give it a lovely, fragrant flavor.

3.   Heat a wok or large frying pan until very hot. Pour in a splash of olive oil and add the onions, garlic and ginger. Fry for a couple of minutes until the onions have softened a little. Drop in the seasoned pieces of beef and stir-fry for a couple of minutes. Add the broccoli spears and fry for a further 2 minutes, stirring all the time.

4.   Pour in the soy sauce and sesame oil. Toss in the pan until everything is well coated. Serve with egg noodles or steamed rice with a wedge of lime and some sliced red chili sprinkled over the top.

NOTE: If you are feeling flash, use fillet steak instead of sirloin in your stir-fry.

Vegan Shepherd's Pie

INGREDIENTS	NUTRITION FACTS (Per Serving)	
600 g Maris Piper potatoes	✓ Calories	389
600 g sweet potatoes	✓ Carbs	51.3g
Sea salt	✓ Sugar	10g
Freshly ground black pepper	✓ Fat	16.3g
40 g dairy-free margarine	✓ Saturates	2.7g
1 onion	✓ Protein	11.2g
2 carrots		
3 cloves of garlic		
2 sticks of celery		
1 tablespoon coriander seeds		
Olive oil		
½ a small bunch of thyme		
350 g chestnut mushrooms		
12 sun-dried tomatoes		
2 tablespoons balsamic vinegar		
Vegan red wine		
100 ml organic vegetable stock		
1 x 400 g tin of lentils		
1 x 400 g tin of chickpeas		
5 sprigs of fresh flat-leaf parsley		
2 sprigs of fresh rosemary		
Zest of 1 lemon		
30 g fresh breadcrumbs		
8 SERVINGS TOTAL TIME 85MINS		

Instructions:

1. Preheat the oven to 200°C/400°F/gas 6.

2. Peel and chop all the potatoes into rough 2cm chunks. Place the Maris Pipers into a large pan of cold salted water over a medium heat. Bring to the boil, then simmer for 10 to 15 minutes, or until tender, adding the sweet potatoes after 5 minutes. Drain and leave to steam dry, then return to the pan with the margarine and a pinch of salt and pepper. Mash until smooth, then set aside.

3. Peel and finely slice the onion, carrots and 2 garlic cloves, then trim and finely slice the celery. Bash the coriander seeds in a pestle and mortar until fine, then add it all to a medium pan over a medium heat with a good splash of olive oil. Pick in the thyme leaves, then cook for around 10 minutes, or until softened.

4. Meanwhile, roughly chop the mushrooms and sun-dried tomatoes. Add to the pan along with the vinegar and 2 tablespoons of the sun-dried tomato oil from the jar. Cook for a further 10 minutes then add a splash of wine, turn up the heat, and allow it to boil and bubble away. Stir in the stock, lentils and chickpeas (juice and all), then leave it to tick away for 5 to 10 minutes, or until slightly thickened and reduced. Pick and roughly chop the parsley leaves, then stir

into the pan. Season to taste, then transfer to a large baking dish (roughly 25cm x 30cm).

5.   Spread the mash over the top, scuffing it up with the back of a spoon. Finely slice the remaining garlic clove, then place into a bowl with the rosemary leaves, lemon zest, breadcrumbs and 1 tablespoon of olive oil. Mix well, sprinkle over the mash, then place in the hot oven for around 10 minutes, or until piping hot through. Place under the grill for a further 2 to 3 minutes, or until golden, then serve with your favorite greens.

Sloppy Joe

INGREDIENTS	NUTRITION FACTS (Per Serving)	
¾ pound quality lean ground beef (10% fat) or turkey	✓ Calories	507
1 yellow onion, peeled and diced	✓ Carbs	52.4g
1 green bell pepper, cored, seeded and diced	✓ Sugar	25.2g
¾ cup tomato puree	✓ Fat	17.9g
2 tablespoons cider vinegar	✓ Saturates	6.5g
1½ tablespoons light brown sugar	✓ Protein	29g
1 tablespoon honey		
2 teaspoons Dijon mustard		
½ teaspoon chili powder		
½ can kidney beans, drained and rinsed		
Freshly ground pepper, to taste		
4 whole wheat hamburger buns or whole wheat wraps		
1 cup shredded lettuce		
4 SERVINGS TOTAL TIME 35MINS		

Instructions:

1. Put a large sauté pan over a medium heat and crumble in the beef or turkey. Fry until the meat starts to brown then add the bell pepper and onion. Continue cooking, stirring occasionally, until the veggies start to soften – this should take around 5 to 10 minutes.

2. When the veggies are tender, add the tomato purée and stir into the meat, then add the vinegar, brown sugar, honey, mustard and chile powder to the pan and give everything a really good stir. Add the beans, season with salt and pepper, then bring to a boil and cook until the sauce is nice and thick.

To serve:

Pile the Sloppy Joe mix onto the bottom of a bun or middle of a wrap, top it with lettuce and close up the sandwich or roll up the wrap.

Serving suggestions:

Delicious served with an Everyday chopped green salad or some Brilliant broccoli.

Summer Fruit, Elderflower & Prosecco Jelly

INGREDIENTS	NUTRITION FACTS (Per Serving)	
8 punnets mixed soft fruit	✓ Calories	144
(blackberries, raspberries,	✓ Carbs	20.3g
strawberries, blueberries)	✓ Sugar	20.3g
4 leaves beef gelatin	✓ Fat	0.4g
140 ml elderflower cordial	✓ Saturates	0.1g
2 heaped tablespoons caster sugar	✓ Protein	2.7g
425 ml Prosecco, chilled		
10 SERVING		
TOTAL TIME 15MINS		

Instructions:

1. First of all, decide whether you want to make one big jelly or small individual ones. If you are making a big one, it's a good idea to line the bowl with clingfilm first. Put your ripe fruit into your mould or moulds and refrigerate.

2. Put your gelatine leaves into a bowl with a little cold water to soak for a minute, then drain and add the gelatine back to the bowl with the cordial. Rest above a pan of water over a medium heat and stir constantly until the gelatine and cordial become a syrup. At this point you can add your sugar, stir till

dissolved, then remove the bowl from the heat and let it sit at room temperature for a minute or so.

3.   Take your fruit and Prosecco out of the fridge. The idea being that your fruit, moulds and Prosecco are all chilled, so the bubbles stay in the jelly when it sets and they fizz in your mouth when you eat it - beautiful! Pour the Prosecco into your cordial mix, and then pour this over your fruit. Some of the fruit might rise to the top, so using your finger, just push the fruit down into the jelly mix so that it is sealed and will then keep well in the fridge. Put back into the fridge for an hour to set.

4.   To serve, dip your mould into a bowl of hot water to loosen the outside of the jelly, then turn it out on to a plate. Great served with a little crème fraîche but just as good on its own.

Pear Sorbet (Sorbetto di pere)

INGREDIENTS	NUTRITION FACTS (Per Serving)		
200 g caster sugar	✓	Calories	213
200 ml water	✓	Carbs	49.8g
1 kg soft pears, peeled,	✓	Sugar	49.8g
quartered and cores removed	✓	Fat	0.2g
Juice and zest of 1 lemon	✓	Saturates	0.0g
55 ml grappa, or to taste	✓	Protein	0.7g
6 SERVINGS			
TOTAL TIME 25MINS			

Instructions:

1. First of all put the sugar and water into a pan on the hob. Bring to the boil, then reduce the heat and simmer for 3 minutes.

2. Add your quartered pears and, unless they're super soft, continue to simmer for 5 minutes. Remove from the heat, leave to one side for 5 minutes, then add the lemon juice (minus the pips) and zest.

3. Pour everything into a food processor and whiz to a purée, then push the mixture through a coarse sieve into the dish in which you want to serve it.

4. Add the grappa, give it a good stir, and taste. The grappa shouldn't be overbearing or too powerful – it should be subtle and should work well with the pears. However, different brands do vary in strength and flavour, so add to taste. (This isn't an excuse to add the whole bottle, though, because if you use too much alcohol the sorbet won't freeze.)

5. Put the dish into the freezer and whisk it up with a fork every half-hour – you'll see it becoming pale in color. After a couple of hours it will be ready. The texture should be nice and scoop-able.

6. Delicious served with ventagli or other delicate crunchy biscuits.

Toxin Less Recipes

This elimination resets your testosterone level to normal. It also supports the reset of estrogen, insulin, leptin and thyroid. Killing a lot of birds with one hormone reset, ey?

Clean Eating Banana Muesli

INGREDIENTS
1/4 cup raw, old fashion oats
1/4 cup raw almonds
1 tbsp chia seeds
1/2 medium banana
1/4 cup fat-free, soy milk or almond milk
1 SERVING
TOTAL TIME 5MINS

Instructions:

1.   Combine all ingredients in a bowl and serve!

Smashed Avocado Toast

INGREDIENTS
2 small slices gluten-free & whole
grain or sprouted grain bread
1 small or 1/2 large ripe avocado,
about 2 tablespoons per slice
1 pinch Real Salt or natural garlic sea salt
Optional: sprinkle of your favorite chili flakes
2 SERVINGS
TOTAL TIME 10MINS

Instructions:

E R I E   C H I L D S

2.   Lightly toast the bread.

3.   While the bread is toasting, mash the avocado with the salt using a fork.

4.   Spread the avocado on warm toast then sprinkle with chili flakes if you're using and enjoy.

5.   Every once in a while I'll add a drizzle of a high-quality extra virgin olive oil for added flavor.

Gluten Free Pasta Salad

INGREDIENTS	NUTRITION FACTS (Per Serving)		
16 ounces brown rice pasta	✓	Calories	318.5
4 ounces sun-dried	✓	Calories from Fat 232	73%
tomatoes (chopped)	✓	Total Fat 25.8g	39%
1/2 cup pine nuts (toasted)	✓	Saturated Fat 6.8g	33%
4 ounces feta cheese (crumbled)	✓	Cholesterol 31.2mg	10%
1/4 cup fresh basil (chopped)	✓	Sodium 1033.6mg	43%
2 garlic cloves (minced)	✓	Total Carbs 16.4g	5%
1/2 red bell pepper (finely diced)	✓	Dietary Fiber 3.4g	13%
1/2 red onion (finely diced)	✓	Sugars 9.8g	39%
4 ounces hard Italian	✓	Protein 9.9g	19%
salami (small cubed)			
1 green onion (chopped)			
1/2 teaspoon salt			
1/2 teaspoon pepper			
1 1/2 teaspoons oregano			
1/4 cup extra virgin olive oil			
1/4 cup lemon juice			
6-8 SERVINGS			
TOTAL TIME 30MINS			

Instructions:

1. Cook pasta according to package directions (about 10 minutes in boiling water until al dente).

2. Whisk together olive oil, lemon juice, salt, pepper, oregano and set aside.

3.   Cool pasta in cold water and drain well.

4.   Add remaining ingredients to a large bowl and mix well.

5.   Add olive oil mixture and mix well.

6.   Serve immediately or let marinate overnight in tight container.

NOTE: To toast the pine nuts, pre-heat a skillet over medium heat. Add pine nuts and stir occasionally until lightly browned.

French Potato Salad

INGREDIENTS	NUTRITION FACTS (Per Serving)		
1 lb small white potatoes	✓	Calories	486.4
1 lb small red potato	✓	Calories from Fat 306	63%
2 tablespoons good	✓	Total Fat 34.1g	52%
dry white wine	✓	Saturated Fat 4.8g	23%
2 tablespoons chicken stock	✓	Cholesterol 0.2mg	0%
3 tablespoons white	✓	Sodium 1779mg	74%
balsamic vinegar	✓	Total Carbohydrate 41.1g	13%
½ teaspoon Dijon mustard	✓	Dietary Fiber 5.4g	21%
1 tablespoon kosher salt	✓	Sugars 2.1g	8%
¾ teaspoon fresh ground pepper	✓	Protein 5.1g	10%
10 tablespoons olive oil			
¼ cup minced green onion			
(white and green parts)			
2 tablespoons minced fresh dill			
2 tablespoons minced parsley			
2 tablespoons chiffonade			
fresh basil leaves			
4-6 SERVINGS			
TOTAL TIME 20MINS			

Instructions:

1. Cut potatoes in half, quarters if they are larger.

2. Steam until cooked--can pierce easily with fork (can boil if you prefer).

3.   Drain in colander and place a towel over the potatoes to allow them to steam for 10 more minutes.

4.   Place in medium bowl and toss gently with the wine and chicken stock.

5.   Allow the liquids to soak into the warm potatoes before proceeding.

6.   Combine the mustard, vinegar, salt, pepper and slowly whisk in the olive oil to make an emulsion.

7.   Add the vinegarette to the potatoes.

8.   Add the green onions, dill, parsley, and basil.

9.   Serve warm or at room temperature.

Vegetable Lentil Stew

INGREDIENTS	NUTRITION FACTS (Per Serving)		
2 cups dry lentils	✓	Calories	570.4
3⁄4 cup uncooked brown rice	✓	Calories from Fat 24	4%
1 (28 ounce) can tomatoes,	✓	Total Fat 2.8g	4%
undrained and chopped	✓	Saturated Fat 0.5g	2%
1 (48 ounce) can tomato juice	✓	Cholesterol 0mg	0%
4 cups water	✓	Sodium 837.1mg	34%
4 -5 cloves garlic, minced	✓	Total Carbs 112.5g	37%
1 large onion, chopped	✓	Dietary Fiber 32.8g	131%
3 celery ribs, sliced	✓	Sugars 21.9g	87%
4 carrots, sliced	✓	Protein 29.2g	58%
1 bay leaf			
2 teaspoons dried basil			
2 teaspoons dried oregano			
2 teaspoons dried thyme			
1 teaspoon pepper			
3 tablespoons chopped			
fresh parsley			
1 zucchini, chopped			
2 medium potatoes,			
peeled and chopped			
2 tablespoons lemon juice			
1 teaspoon dry mustard			
Salt			
1 SERVING			
TOTAL TIME 140MINS			

Instructions:

1. In a large Dutch oven, mix together the first 15 ingredients.

2. Bring to a boil; reduce heat to low and simmer until rice and lentils are tender, about 1 hour.

3. Add more water or tomato juice if necessary.

4. Stir in the remaining ingredients.

5. Cover and continue cooking until vegetables are tender, usually 1 hour.

Steamed Ginger Fish & Vegetables

INGREDIENTS	NUTRITION FACTS (Per Serving)		
200 g fresh white fish fillets	✓	Calories	368.2
3⁄4 cup cooked rice	✓	Calories from Fat 26	7%
2 teaspoons grated fresh ginger	✓	Total Fat 2.9g	4%
1 tablespoon fresh lemon juice	✓	Saturated Fat 0.6g	2%
Mixed vegetables,	✓	Cholesterol 134mg	44%
steamed to serve	✓	Sodium 144.7mg	6%
	✓	Total Carbohydrate 41.9g	13%
	✓	Dietary Fiber 0.6g	2%
1 SERVING	✓	Sugars 0.4g	1%
TOTAL TIME 30MINS	✓	Protein 40.1g	80%

Instructions:

1. Place a bamboo basket over a saucepan of boiling water.

NOTE: A metal steamer is a good alternative if a bamboo steamer is not available.

2. Line base with baking paper and top with fish.

3. Sprinkle with ginger and lemon juice.

4. Cover and steam for 7 minutes or until fish is cooked depending on how thick the fish is.

5. Serve with vegetables & rice.

No Bake Apple Crumble

INGREDIENTS	NUTRITION FACTS (Per Serving)		
8 apples, peeled and chopped	✓	Calories	306.2
1 cup raisins, soaked and drained	✓	Calories from Fat 140	46%
1 teaspoon cinnamon	✓	Total Fat 15.6g	24%
1/4 teaspoon nutmeg	✓	Saturated Fat 1.5g	7%
2 tablespoons lemon juice	✓	Cholesterol 0mg	0%
2 cups walnuts	✓	Sodium 32.8mg	1%
1 cup pitted dates	✓	Total Carbohydrate 44g	14%
1 teaspoon cinnamon	✓	Dietary Fiber 6.4g	25%
1/8 teaspoon salt	✓	Sugars 32g	128%
	✓	Protein 4.8g	9%
10 SERVINGS TOTAL TIME 20MINS			

Instructions:

1. To make filling, in a food processor, place 2 apples with raisins, cinnamon and nutmeg, process until smooth.

2. In a bowl place remaining chopped apples and toss with lemon juice.

3. Pour pureed filling mixture over top, mix well.

4. Spoon apple mixture into a med sized lasagna pan and set aside.

5. For crumble, in a food processor, pulse walnuts, dates, cinnamon and salt until coarsely ground.

6. Do not over mix.

7. Crumble the mixture over the apples with your hands and press lightly.

8. Serve immediately or let marinate for a few hours for extra flavor.

Raw Banana Pudding

INGREDIENTS	NUTRITION FACTS (Per Serving)		
2 bananas, peeled	✓	Calories	370.8
½ an avocado, peeled and seeded	✓	Calories from Fat 139	38%
Raw pistachios, chopped (garnish)	✓	Total Fat 15.5g	23%
	✓	Saturated Fat 2.4g	12%
1-2 SERVINGS	✓	Cholesterol 0mg	0%
TOTAL TIME 10MINS	✓	Sodium 9.4mg	0%
	✓	Total Carbohydrate 62.5g	20%
	✓	Dietary Fiber 12.9g	51%
	✓	Sugars 29.5g	118%
	✓	Protein 4.6g	9%

Instructions:

1. Blend banana and avocado until smooth and fluffy.

2. Chill 'til ready to serve, at which time top with pistachios as a garnish.

Sweet Potato Soup

INGREDIENTS	NUTRITION FACTS (Per Serving)		
32 ounces carrot juice (fresh)	✓	Calories	220
1 medium sweet potato	✓	Calories from Fat 69	32%
(cubed, peeled)	✓	Total Fat 7.8g	11%
4 dates, pitted	✓	Saturated Fat 1.1g	5%
1 avocado (scooped out)	✓	Cholesterol 0mg	0%
3 dashes pumpkin pie spice	✓	Sodium 87.9mg	3%
	✓	Total Carbohydrate 37.4g	12%
	✓	Dietary Fiber 6.8g	27%
4-5 SERVINGS	✓	Sugars 15.1g	60%
TOTAL TIME 15MINS	✓	Protein 3.9g	7%

Instructions:

1. Blend until smooth.

2. Enjoy as much as you like!

Vitality Soup

INGREDIENTS	NUTRITION FACTS (Per Serving)		
1 cup distilled water	✓	Calories	189.6
1⁄2 cup fresh orange juice	✓	Calories from Fat 71	38%
1⁄4 cup fresh lemon juice	✓	Total Fat 7.9g	12%
6 ounces greens	✓	Saturated Fat 1.2g	5%
(spinach, kale, etc.)	✓	Cholesterol 0mg	0%
1 medium apple,	✓	Sodium 1172.8mg	48%
quartered and cored	✓	Total Carbohydrate 31.9g	10%
1⁄2-1 medium avocado,	✓	Dietary Fiber 6.8g	27%
quartered, peeled and pitted	✓	Sugars 18.5g	73%
1 cucumber, chopped	✓	Protein 3g	6%
1 garlic clove, crushed			
1 green onion, chopped			
1⁄4habanero pepper (optional)			
1⁄8-1⁄4 teaspoon ground kelp or			
1⁄8-1⁄4 teaspoon dulse seaweed			
1 teaspoon sea salt, to taste			
2 SERVINGS			
TOTAL TIME 10MINS			

Instructions:

1.   Combine all ingredients in a blender and puree until smooth. Adjust flavors to taste and serve at room temperature.

Reminders and More

There you have it – all the recipes that you would need for your 21 day reset diet. Just a few reminders though:

- Remember that you can add your own recipes to the mix. Don't be scared to just go online and Google for recipes that you find appetizing. Again, these recipes are just guides for you to follow.

- I've included a good mix of recipes into this book. Some are easy to do, some have a little bit of difficulty to them *(intermediate level of cooking)*. This is why I encourage you to bring a bit of your flavor to the recipes. It's your diet anyway, right?

- Don't underestimate the whole program. It's surprising how much time it takes to prepare a meal so make sure that you do all the necessary steps to keep yourself going – reminders, charts, planners and etc. If you manage your time well, prepping the dishes and cooking them will be a cinch.

- Never mind about counting the calories. Did I just say that? Yes. Please put away your calorie counter because…well, that's a whole other topic on its own but I've found a couple of helpful resources for you to read online:

- o   MarishRiver.com

- o   Prevention.com

- o   PaleoLeap.com

- o   MindBodyGreen.com

- o   EvidenceMag.com

Chapter 6

EATING AFTER HORMONE RESET

When you've already reached this point, it means that you may have already finished your 21 days! Congratulations! If you're just reading ahead, don't worry; you'll finish your 21 soon enough – hang in there!

After doing your 21 day hormone reset, you're going to prepare yourself for reentry. This means that you need to incorporate the foods that you were eating before resetting your hormones. This is not a bad thing at all since you've experienced the changes that your body has felt for 21 days. The process may have already taught you to listen to your body. You'll be able to tell what type of food causes a certain reaction and what doesn't.

Do your reentry slowly and refrain from binging on the types of food you miss the most. Don't overdose your body just to cause your hormones to go out of whack again.

Chapter 7

LIFE AFTER HORMONE RESET

Now, it's time to assess how your reset has affected you. Hopefully, you've kept a journal of your journey. If you did, check back on the metrics that you had before doing your reset. Check each one and then notice the difference. You may also notice how you feel, overall. How has the reset affected your mood? Do you still have mood swings? These are the kinds of questions that you should be asking yourself.

Now that you've done your reset, you need to maintain the level that your hormones are on, right? Instead of living your life the way you did before, maintain the lifestyle as well as the eating habits that you have right now. If you've trained yourself to just take in smoothies in the morning, go ahead and do it. You've probably already made a habit of it so why change it now that you're not on a reset anymore?

Chapter 8

WORDS OF WISDOM

Hi there. I hope that you found this book helpful. I just wanted to add this section in so I can sneak in a few words about resetting hormones.

The struggle with weight is real! No matter what diet or exercise we do, we always find it difficult to lose a certain amount of weight given the little amount of time *(and sometimes resources)* that we have every day. Am I preaching to the congregation yet? If I hit a note, that's because I've gone through it myself. I know how difficult it is to lose weight if you don't even have time to exercise or if you don't have enough resources to prepare and eat the right kind of food.

This is why I made the program customizable. I want you to add in what you can contribute. You don't have to, strictly, follow the recipes I stated here. Make it your own. As for exercising, you can do without it for this program but I encourage you to have 30mins of moving every day. It could be basic stretches, walking, jogging or what have you. Just make sure that you move your body 30mins a day.

Also, don't be intimidated by success stories you read online saying that the program worked for them and they lost 1million pounds in just 3 weeks *(an exaggeration, of course)*. Though we are correcting the same kind of hormones, our body can react differently to the program causing you to lose weight slowly or drastically. Trust the process and trust how your body feels. Go through with it and see if you can note any difference. If you can, that means that something is happening and you just need to keep at it for 21 days.

What I'm saying may sound easy to say but hard to do. That's because it is. This is the hard truth to it. Even if you're moving 30 mins a day and you've found a way to customize the meals to fit your resources, it's still going to take a much of your time and effort but the good news is, there's a pot of gold at the end of the rainbow and I'm really hoping that you find your pit of gold soon!

I wish you the best of luck with your hormone reset!

FAQ

- **Do I need to exercise while on this program?**

  o Not necessarily but you'll get better results when you do exercise. It doesn't have to be an hour of cross fit every day. Like I said earlier, you just have to make sure that your body is moving – stretches will do, basic yoga poses will do, walking to the nearest park will do and jogging for 30 mins will, definitely do.

  o Find an exercise that fits your time. There's no specific exercise requirement, remember that.

- **How will I be feeling while on the hormone reset?**

  o The hormone reset will be managing your hormones so it's highly likely that your mood swings and your cravings will be under control. How you feel will be entirely up to how your body is reacting. It's different from one individual to another.

- **How much weight will I lose?**

  o I've mentioned this earlier. This will, again, depend on how your body reacts to the program. You can lose as much as 15lbs in just 3 weeks but, another scenario is that, you may not lose much at all.

  o DON'T PANIC! My advice is to keep at it so you can, thoroughly, reset your hormones and then you can measure your metrics right after to really tell if it was effective or not. You might just be surprised about what you'll discover with your results!

- **What should I do if I have cravings?**

  o Remember when I said that you need to exercise your will power at least for the first few days? It's no-negotiable. If you're experiencing cravings, simply don't give in to them. Instead, replace them with something that you CAN eat during your hormone reset. Snack on something healthy that doesn't go beyond what's inhibited.

- **Will I gain weight after I do the program?**

    o   It's not impossible, let me tell you that. The thought of reentry after 21 days of diet restrictions is very heavenly. Do go overboard as you may cause one or two hormonal imbalances. Then, you're back to ground zero if this happens and this means that you're probably going to gain back the weight you lost.

- **Is the program safe to do?**

    o   Yes it is. If you're feeling extra anxious about it, go and check with your doctor or with your nutritionist. Nonetheless, please remember that this program is just like any diet out there *(like the paleo diet or gluten free diet as you may notice with the recipes)*. The main difference is it's merely geared towards resetting hormones and it's not just about eating well and losing weight.

Check Out All My Other BEST SELLING BOOKS Below!

---

http://www.amazon.com/Valerie-Childs/e/B00VVS8TYO

You'll Find 16+ Books on Health, Nutrition, Cooking and even Gardening!

Here are a few quick titles…

- Unleash the Power of the Paleo Diet

- Paleo Slow Cooker

- Green Smoothie Cleanse

- Sugar Detox

- Green Smoothie Cleanse

- The Ultimate Guide to Gardening (5 in 1 Combo Set)

- AND MANY, MANY MORE!

Check Out My BEST SELLING BOOKS HERE -> http://

www.amazon.com/Valerie-Childs/e/B00VVS8TYO

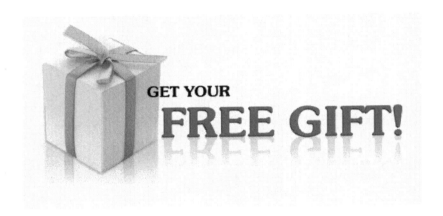

WAIT! – DO YOU LIKE FREE BOOKS?

My **FREE Gift** to You!! As a way to say **Thank You** for downloading my book, I'd like to offer you more **FREE BOOKS!** Each time we release a NEW book, we offer it first to a small number of people as a test - drive. Because of your commitment here in downloading my book, I'd love for you to be a part of this group. You can join easily here → http://smoothieslimdown.com/

Conclusion

Thank you again for downloading this book!

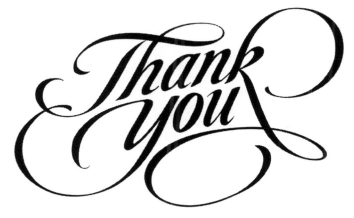

If you enjoyed this book, then I'd like to ask you for a favor, would you be kind enough to leave a review for this book on Amazon? It'd be greatly appreciated!

Help us better serve you by sending questions or comments to greatreadspublishing@gmail.com - Thank you!

26026871R00092

Made in the USA
Middletown, DE
17 November 2015